MW00333917

DASH Diet Cookbook for Beginners

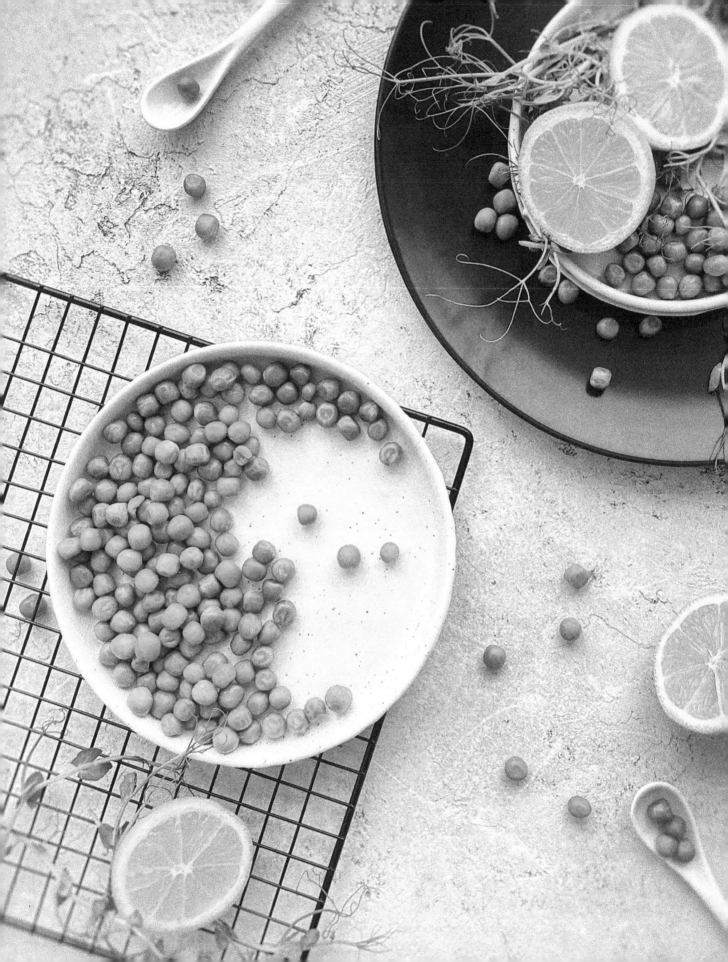

DASH DIET
COOKBOOK
FOR BEGINNERS

Healthy and Low-Sodium Recipes with 21-Day Meal Plan to Lower
Blood Pressure and Improve Your Health

Shirley Deangelo

Copyright© 2021 By Shirley Deangelo All Rights Reserved

This book is copyright protected. It is only for personal use. You cannot amend, distribute, sell, use, quote or paraphrase any part of the content within this book, without the consent of the author or publisher.

Under no circumstances will any blame or legal responsibility be held against the publisher, or author, for any damages, reparation, or monetary loss due to the information contained within this book, either directly or indirectly.

Disclaimer Notice:Please note the information contained within this document is for educational and entertainment purposes only. All effort has been executed to present accurate, up to date, reliable, complete information. No warranties of any kind are declared or implied. Readers acknowledge that the author is not engaged in the rendering of legal, financial, medical or professional advice. The content within this book has been derived from various sources. Please consult a licensed professional before attempting any techniques outlined in this book.

By reading this document, the reader agrees that under no circumstances is the author responsible for any losses, direct or indirect, that are incurred as a result of the use of the information contained within this document, including, but not limited to, errors, omissions, or inaccuracies.

CONTENT

Introduction 1

Chapter 1 The Basics of the DASH Diet   2

Chapter 2 Breakfasts and Smoothies   13

Chapter 3 Salads, Soups, and Sandwiches   29

Chapter 4 Vegetarian and Vegan Mains   48

Chapter 5 Poultry and Fish 68

Chapter 6 Beef and Pork   85

Chapter 7 Snacks, Sides, and Desserts   97

Chapter 8 Broths, Condiments, and Sauces   113

Appendix 1 Measurement Conversion Chart 123

Appendix 2 Measurement Conversion Chart 125

Appendix 3 The Dirty Dozen and Clean Fifteen   126

Appendix 4 Recipe Index   127

References   128

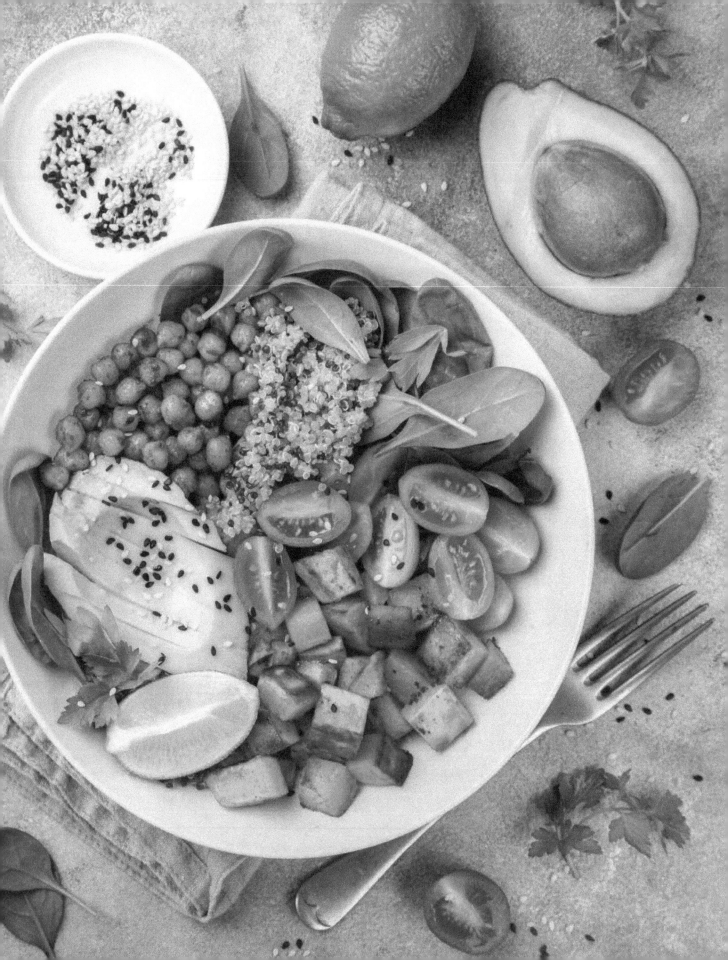

Introduction

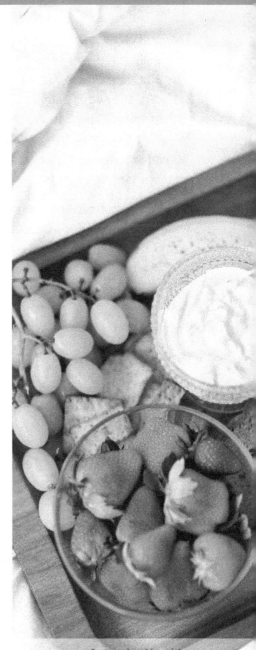

When you are dealing with hypertension, you may find yourself in a constant battle of keeping your blood pressure at decent levels. You might even take medicine to keep things under control, but there is only so much that medicine can do for you. You need to be able to take care of your own body, to help it function in the manner that it was supposed to.

Maybe you have always had very high blood pressure. Maybe you just have the occasional spikes above the average. No matter the case, there is one diet that was made with this exact condition in mind. And this is the DASH diet. It tells you exactly what you should and should not eat so that your blood pressure goes back to its normal level.

Chapter 1 The Basics of the DASH Diet

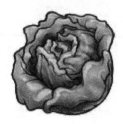

The DASH diet isn't that difficult to follow, particularly when you already have a good idea of the products that you can eat. The only matter that you need to be careful about is the number of servings. The basic idea is more about the foods that you can eat, not necessarily cutting out food.

For example, the DASH diet may easily have you consuming about 2,000 calories a day, although this depends on your age, your activity level, and other variables. The basis of this diet is to have you eating healthy so that you promote weight loss and give your body the necessary nutrients.

Aside from the standard DASH diet, there is also a lower-sodium version of it. This means that you can choose the plan that is most appropriate for your needs (i.e., the higher your average blood pressure, the lower the sodium levels should be). **Here is how much you will have to consume:**

- 2,300 mg of sodium per day for the standard DASH diet

- 1,500 mg of sodium per day for the lower sodium DASH diet

Both DASH diet options have the purpose of reducing your daily sodium intake. The average American ingests around 3,400 mg of sodium every day, and the purpose of the DASH diet is to keep it under 2,300 per day. This will lower your blood pressure along with allowing you to eat healthy foods.

The DASH diet was made to be a lifestyle rather than a manner to lose weight. With that in mind, if your body accommodates properly to the DASH diet, then you will bring it in a certain balance and a state that it was naturally supposed to be in.

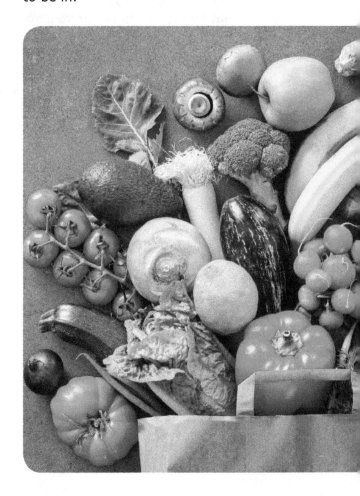

What Is the DASH Diet?

The DASH Diet stands for Dietary Approach to Stop Hypertension. To put it simply, this diet has the purpose of doing exactly that: stopping or preventing hypertension. It focuses on fruits and veggies, healthy fats, low-fat dairy, lean protein, and whole grains.

The DASH diet is high in certain nutrients such as calcium, magnesium, potassium, and fiber while being low in trans fats, saturated fats, and sodium. It is a diet that has been scientifically proven to reduce instances of hypertension, without any side effects.

With that in mind, for the DASH diet to work, people should make certain changes in their lifestyle. Things such as drinking enough water or sticking to an exercise plan should also be adhered to. You also have a variety of recipes that can help make matters easier, which you can find out about in my DASH diet cookbook. Also, remember that with the DASH diet, you should always discuss matters closely with your physician.

Benefits of the DASH Diet

The DASH diet comes with various benefits that you may be able to reap, the most popular ones being a lowered blood pressure and potential weight loss that we'll touch upon a bit later. These potential benefits should tell you whether this diet is right for you or not. It should also help you differentiate it from many other diets on the market. Here is what you may expect from it:

Stronger Bones

The calcium and magnesium part of the DASH diet is meant to lower your blood pressure. However, this also helps ensure that your bones remain in peak shape. The calcium will strengthen your bones, and the magnesium will ensure that it sticks properly.

By following this diet, those who often have problems with arthritis and other similar conditions might find relief. Not to mention that it will protect your bones in the event of any incident occurring. Supplements are technically safe, but it's always a good idea to get your calcium intake through proper nutrition.

Healthier Heart

As the DASH diet keeps your blood pressure at lower levels, it will also protect your heart from a variety of conditions. The potassium you take from the DASH diet will also lower the risk of cardiac arrest and other cardiovascular conditions. It is a more convenient alternative to taking potassium supplements. Without the correct supervision, these supplements can cause various problems as a result of an overdose.

Decreased Risk of Diabetes

Some studies show that by following the DASH diet, you also put yourself at a lower risk for Type 2 Diabetes. Plus, it is believed that it can improve your insulin resistance. In the end, if you know you are predisposed to developing diabetes, the DASH diet can help you steer clear of these dangers.

Not Restrictive

It depends on their purpose, but most diets can end up being quite restrictive. However, the DASH diet is not that restrictive. In fact, it is quite flexible. The calorie intake can be accommodated to a variety of activity levels and ages, which means that it is not a diet in which you have to starve yourself.

To put it in simple terms, it is a plan that allows you to remain satiated but switches some of the ingredients so that you may stay healthy. Plus, there are a few creative recipes that you may try, which can help you enjoy your meals while sticking to your plan. You may find some ideas for recipes in my DASH diet cookbook.

Nutritious

Unlike a variety of other diets, this one doesn't deprive you of the nutrients that you need. It just directs you towards healthier containers of those nutrients, ensuring that your blood pressure stays low. The diet does not necessarily focus on cutting off calories, but rather on switching your body towards a healthier lifestyle.

Prevents Gout

People with gout often experience heightened serum uric acid levels, leading to inflammation throughout their whole body. Often, this causes higher blood pressure, leading to a variety of other conditions.

DASH diet has proven to be able to lower those serum uric acid levels, preventing this inflammatory condition. People with gout are often known to have high blood pressure. So, by taking away the problem posed by gout, you are also lowering your blood pressure.

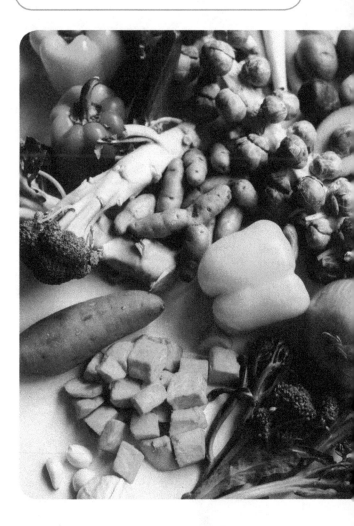

Weight Loss and DASH Diet

As you can see, the DASH is great if you want to maintain a healthy lifestyle, and while it was not specifically tailored for weight loss, it can still be adjusted for you to reach that goal.

The primary purpose of the DASH plan is to bring your blood pressure to proper numbers, to make you feel healthier, and to reduce your hypertension. It doesn't feature any quick weight loss phases (something very common with most diets), and rather than focusing on lost pounds, it puts the emphasis on better general well-being.

With that in mind, the fact that it focuses mostly on healthy ingredients may as well help you lose weight. Since you are no longer ingesting as much sodium, your body will not retain as much water, which can eventually let you lose weight and shed off that unsightly cellulite.

Plus, you won't be consuming as many sweets (if any) with the DASH diet, and since you have to let go of sodium, you need to say goodbye to processed foods as well. These foods are packed with preservatives, a form of sodium that will increase your blood pressure. If your previous diet used to include these kinds of foods, then your system will eventually pick on the new eating plan and allow you to shed the extra weight.

The DASH diet was made so that its followers would ingest somewhere around 2,000 calories per day (depending on their build and activity level). However, this may also be adjusted so that you can find yourself in a calorie deficit and lose weight.

Blood Pressure and DASH Diet

Blood pressure is described as the force that is placed upon your organs and blood vessels as your blood is passing through them. Blood pressure is broken down into two different types (or numbers):

- Systolic pressure, which is the blood vessel pressure when your heart is giving a beat.

- Diastolic pressure, which is the blood vessel pressure between your heartbeats (i.e., when your heart is resting).

The normal blood pressure for an adult is as follows:

- Below 120 mmHg for systolic pressure

- Below 80 mmHg for diastolic pressure

In other words, for someone to have what's considered to be normal blood pressure, it should be somewhere around the lines of 120/80 (systolic pressure is always written above diastolic pressure). However, if someone registers a 140/80 blood pressure, then that number is considered to be within the high ranks.

Blood pressure is often affected by the type of nutrients you ingest, good and bad. For example, sodium is known to raise your blood pressure, which is why doctors recommend that you stay away from processed food and salt when dealing with high blood pressure. On the other hand, certain ingredients specific to the DASH diet can also lower blood pressure, namely calcium, potassium, and magnesium.

The DASH diet demonstrates that it can lower blood pressure in both healthy people and those suffering from high blood pressure. This happened regardless of whether they lost weight or reduced their salt intake.

The results were most impressive among those who already had high blood pressure, reducing 12 mmHg off the systolic scale and 5 mmHg off the diastolic one. In normal patients without blood pressure issues, the blood pressure was reduced by 4 mmHg by the systolic scale and 2 mmHg by the diastolic one.

If salt intake is diminished during the DASH diet, blood pressure is reduced even more, particularly among those that already had high blood pressure, to begin with. However, bear in mind that lower blood pressure does not put you at a lower risk for a heart condition. Very low blood pressure can lead to other issues, which is why you may want to maintain it within the normal scale.

Does It Work for Everyone?

Many people may benefit from the DASH diet, but even so, the best results were seen in individuals that already have high blood pressure. With that in mind, if your blood pressure is within normal levels, the chances are that you may not see any significant results.

Some doctors also suggest that several categories of people should exercise caution when undergoing the DASH diet. While the diet is safe and healthy for most people, those who have chronic liver disease, kidney disease, or those who have been prescribed renin-angiotensin-aldosterone system (RAAS) inhibitors should be careful. Ideally, discussions with your physician should be due.

Certain modifications of the DASH diet may also be necessary in case the person has chronic heart failure, lactose intolerance, Mellitus type 2, and celiac disease. This is why you may want to keep in touch with your healthcare provider, to be certain that the diet is your best choice. Depending on the circumstances, you may as well need to make some modifications to the diet.

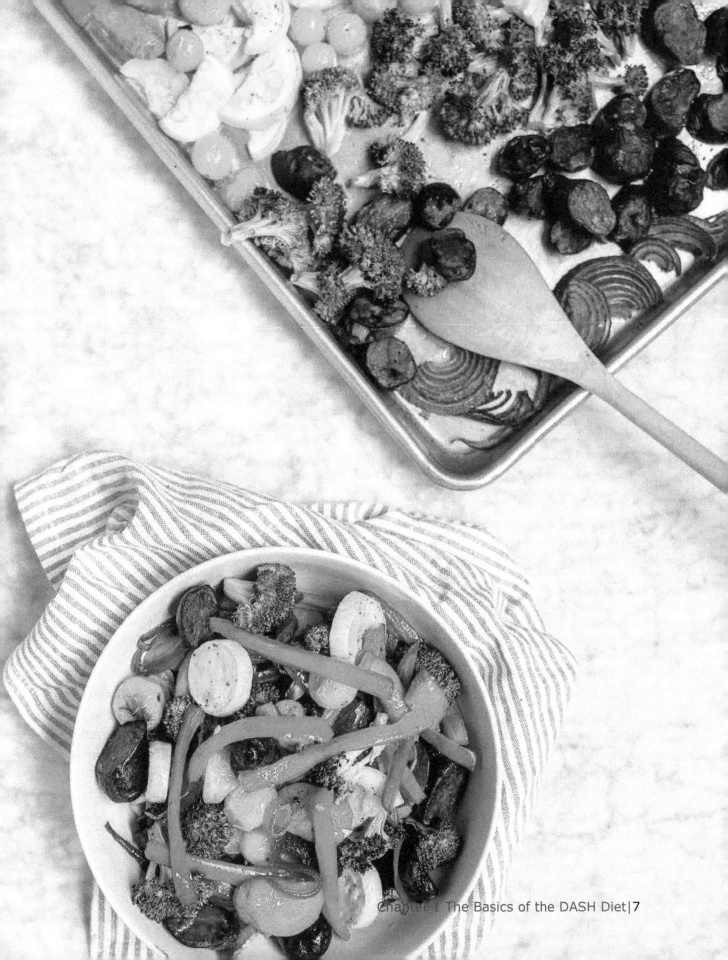

What to Eat on DASH Diet?

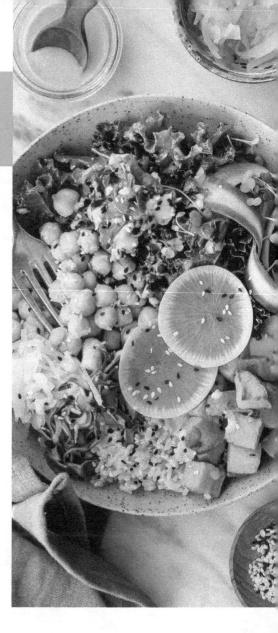

Both DASH diet versions, no matter if you are going for the standard or the lower sodium option, include pretty much the same types of vegetables. The only difference is in the quantities and number of servings.

The DASH diet is quite variable, as you can eat almost anything you want aside from processed, fatty meat and sugary food (although sweets are still allowed in small amounts, and the same thing goes for red meat).

With that in mind, here are the foods that you may eat during the DASH diet, along with the recommended servings per day for an average 2,000 calorie diet. You're not going to eat from all of them, but you may choose which ones you want that day, as long as you do not go over the daily serving size.

You may adjust them according to your desired calorie intake, but you may still want to discuss matters with your healthcare provider. Starving yourself to lose weight is not an option either.

1. Grains (6-8 servings a day)

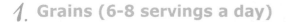

During the DASH diet, grains should be an important part of your meals. Here, you have plenty of options, including pasta, rice, and cereal. Focus on whole grain rather than the refined kind, as it has more nutrients. Also, since grains are naturally very low in fats, avoid putting them in dishes that include cream, butter, and sauces.

2. Vegetables (4-8 servings a day)

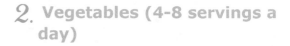

Vegetables such as carrots, tomatoes, sweet potatoes, broccoli, greens, and other veggies are packed with a variety of nutrients. Not only are they high in vitamins and fiber, but they are also rich in magnesium and potassium, the centerpieces of the DASH diet.

3. Fruits (4-5 servings a day)

Except for coconut, fruits are very low in fat and make for great snacks. Plus, they are rich in magnesium, potassium, and fiber, but whenever possible, you might also want to consume them together with the edible peel. Canned fruit is also acceptable, but make sure it doesn't have sugar.

4. Dairy (2-3 servings a day)

Yogurt, milk, cheese, and other dairy products are a great source of calcium, another centerpiece of the DASH diet. However, make sure that you go for low-fat or even fat-free options. This applies mostly to cheese, as the high-fat ones are often packed with sodium.

5. Lean Meat, Fish and Poultry (6 one-ounce servings or less a day)

Meat is packed with B vitamins, protein, zinc, and iron. You may want to focus on lean meat and healthy fish, and you may also want to make sure you trim the skin away.

6. Legumes, Seeds, and Nuts (4-5 servings a week)

Now and again, you may add sunflower seeds, almonds, kidney beans, peas, lentils, and other foods from this category in your diet. They are high in potassium, magnesium, and protein, making them a great choice. However, since they are high in fat, you should make sure you only consume them a few times a week.

7. Fats and Oils (2-3 servings a day)

Fat is necessary for you to absorb the vitamins, but too much of it increases the risk of heart disease. This is why you should get at most 30% of your calories from fat, and make sure those fats are monounsaturated.

8. Sweets (5 servings a week or fewer)

While you don't have to say goodbye entirely to sweets, you might want to keep them under 5 servings a week. Plus, when you DO consume them, make sure they are as low fat as possible. Some good examples can be sorbet, low-fat cookies, and fruit ices. You can find more ideas in my DASH diet cookbook.

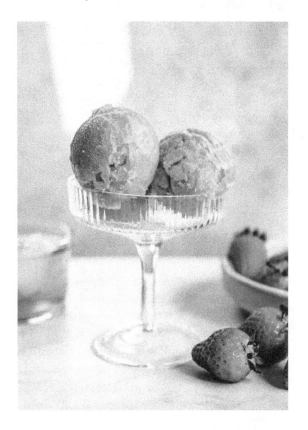

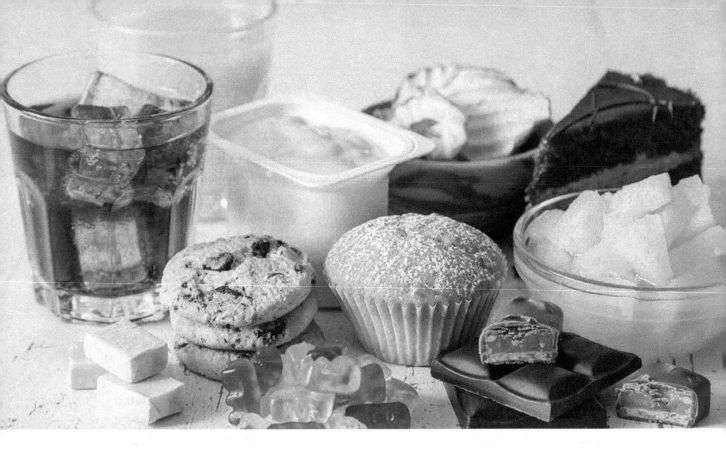

What Foods and Drinks Should Be Avoided?

Certain foods and drinks should also be avoided when you are following the DASH diet. Ideally, **you should steer clear of foods that are packed in sugar, salt, and high fat such as:**

- Cookies
- Candy
- Chips
- Sodas
- Salted nuts
- Pastries
- Sugary beverages
- Snacks
- Meat dishes
- Soups
- Pizza
- Salad dressings
- Rice dishes
- Prepackaged pasta
- High-fat cheese
- Cured meats and cold cuts
- Rolls and bread
- Sauces and gravies
- Sandwiches

Salt substitutes will help you improve the taste of certain dishes and will often come with a high concentration of potassium. This can help lower your blood pressure even further.

FAQs on DASH Diet

Can I have eggs on a DASH diet?

There is a myth going around that eggs raise your cholesterol levels, and therefore, your blood pressure. That being said, with the DASH diet, you are also encouraged to consume lean protein, something that eggs are very rich in. This is why they are a great addition to your DASH diet.

Is it difficult to follow a DASH diet?

It's very easy to follow the DASH diet, as the ingredients are available at every grocery store. The only issue is that since processed food is not allowed, you need to cook things yourself. You can find some good ideas by going through my DASH diet cookbook.

Is exercise necessary while following the DASH diet?

While it's not mandatory (you can lower your blood pressure just as well with the diet alone), it does not mean that you shouldn't pair this plan with some moderate exercising. It will help you lose weight more efficiently if that's your goal, and it may also help your blood pressure issues. After all, you'll be losing the fat that's pressing on your organs.

When will I see results?

The DASH diet works quite fast, and usually, people see results within the first two weeks. This will also depend on how efficient you are in sticking to the diet.

Can I follow the DASH diet even if I don't have high blood pressure?

Yes, while this diet was made specifically for those with high blood pressure, this does not mean that someone with normal blood pressure cannot use it. After all, the diet focuses on healthy foods, so it's not lacking in nutrients.

The Bottom Line

The DASH diet can prove very useful for those struggling with hypertension. It can bring your body back on track, ensuring you get your nutrition while watching what you eat. To make things tastier and not feel like you are on a diet, you may want to check my DASH diet cookbook and prepare some delicious recipes for your next meal.

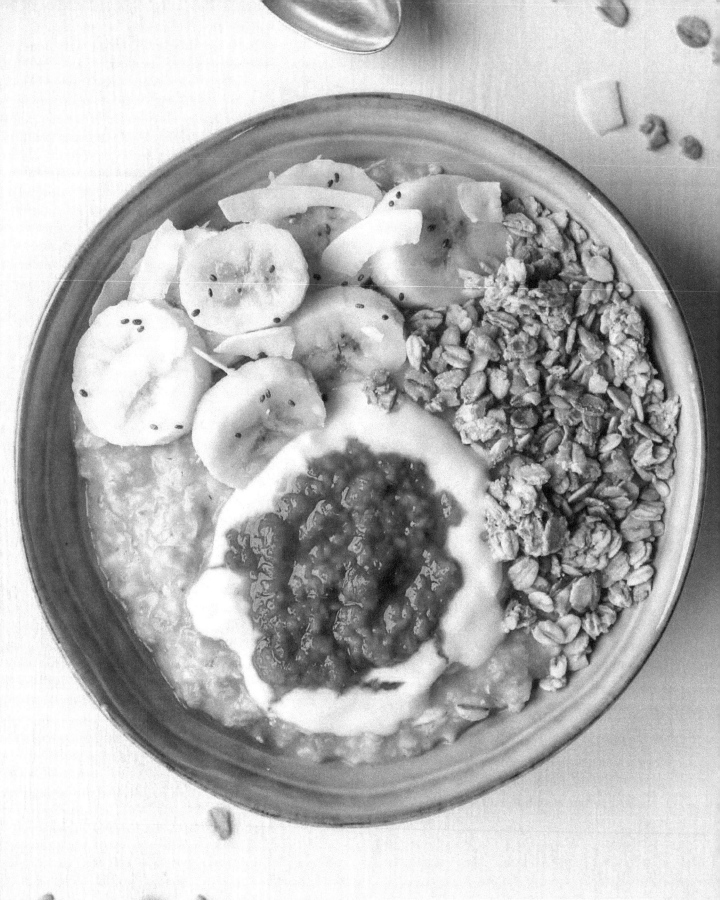

2 BREAKFASTS AND SMOOTHIES

14 Apricot-Banana Breakfast Barley

15 Blueberry-Oatmeal Muffin in a Mug

16 Creamy Peach Quinoa

17 Banana-Almond Pancakes for One

18 High-Protein Apple Carrot Hemp Muffins

19 Egg and Vegetable Breakfast Mug

20 Greek Yogurt Oat Pancakes

21 Sweet Potato and Black Bean Hash

22 Egg in a "Pepper Hole" with Avocado

23 Greek Breakfast Scramble

24 Strawberry Orange Beet Smoothie

25 Green Apple Pie Protein Smoothie

26 Peach Avocado Smoothie

26 Almond Butter Banana Chocolate Smoothie

27 Morning Glory Smoothie

Apricot-Banana Breakfast Barley

Prep Time: 5 minutes

Cook Time: 30 minutes

Serving: 4

---

1 cup pearl barley, rinsed and drained

1 to 1½ cups fat-free milk or plant-based milk

Pinch of salt

4 dried apricots, finely chopped

1 large banana, sliced

4 teaspoons sliced almonds

Sweetener of choice (optional)

1. In a 4-quart saucepan, combine the barley, 2 cups water, 1 cup of the milk, the salt, apricots, and banana. Bring to a boil over high heat, then reduce the heat to low. Cover and cook until most of the liquid is absorbed, about 30 minutes. Add an additional ½ cup milk, if necessary, to reach desired consistency.

2. Portion into 4 bowls and top with sliced almonds and a sweetener, if desired.

Per Serving
(without the extra ½ cup milk)

calories: 258 | fat: 2g | protein: 8g
carbs: 55g | sugars: 11g | fiber: 9g
sodium: 51mg | cholesterol: 1mg

Blueberry-Oatmeal Muffin in a Mug

Prep Time: 1 minutes

Cook Time: 1 minutes

Serving: 1

½ cup rolled oats

1 egg

2 tablespoons nonfat or low-fat milk

$^1/_3$ cup blueberries

Cooking spray

Optional: no-calorie sweetener of choice

1. Spray a large mug or small ramekin with cooking spray.

2. Add the oats, egg, and milk, and stir to combine. Gently fold in the blueberries.

3. Place in the microwave and cook on high for 1 minute, being careful to watch as it could overflow. If the muffin does not look firm, place back in for 30 seconds at a time.

4. Once ready, flip mug upside down onto a plate, slice, and enjoy.

Per Serving

calories: 259 | fat: 8g | protein: 13g
carbs: 36g | sugars: 8g | fiber: 5g
sodium: 87mg | cholesterol: 187mg

Creamy Peach Quinoa

Prep Time: 5 minutes

Cook Time: 20 minutes

Serving: 4

---

1 cup quinoa, rinsed and drained

2 cups fat-free milk

1 cup finely chopped peaches

½ teaspoon ground cinnamon

Pinch of salt

2 tablespoons chopped walnuts

Sweetener of choice (optional)

1. In a medium saucepan, combine the quinoa, milk, peaches, cinnamon, and salt. Stir to combine, bring to a boil, covered. Reduce the heat to medium-low and cook, covered, until most of the liquid has been absorbed, about 20 minutes.

2. Remove the saucepan from the heat and let stand, covered, 5 minutes. Fluff with a fork.

3. Portion into 4 bowls and top each with ½ tablespoon chopped walnuts and sweetener, if desired.

Per Serving

calories: 245 | fat: 5g | protein: 11g
carbs: 41g | sugars: 10g | fiber: 4g
sodium: 81mg | cholesterol: 293mg

Banana-Almond Pancakes for One

Prep Time: 5 minutes

Cook Time: 3 minutes

Serving: 1

---

1 medium banana, sliced

2 large eggs

2 tablespoons almond meal/flour

2 tablespoons quick oats

1 teaspoon almond butter

½ teaspoon baking powder

¼ cup raspberries, washed and drained

1. In a high-powered blender, combine the banana, eggs, almond meal/flour, oats, almond butter, and baking powder and process until smooth. (Don't worry if the batter seems too thin; the pancakes will cook up perfectly.)

2. Coat a skillet with cooking spray and set over medium heat.

3. Pour the batter in 2-tablespoon amounts onto the pan and let cook for about 1 minute. Flip and cook on the other side until lightly browned and firm, about 1 minute more.

4. Serve topped with fresh berries.

Per Serving

calories: 414 | fat: 21g | protein: 19g

carbs: 43g | sugars: 17g | fiber: 8g

sodium: 146mg | cholesterol: 372mg

High-Protein Apple Carrot Hemp Muffins

1 cup nonfat (0%) plain Greek yogurt

2 cups shredded carrots

4 cups diced unpeeled apples

1½ cups oat flour

½ cup plain high-fiber hemp protein

½ cup granulated no-calorie sweetener

1 tablespoon ground nutmeg

1 teaspoon baking soda

1 teaspoon baking powder

¼ teaspoon salt

½ cup liquid egg whites

1. Preheat the oven to 350ºF (180ºC). Coat 12 cups of a standard muffin tin with cooking spray.

2. In a blender, combine the yogurt, carrots, and apples and blend until it has the consistency of applesauce.

3. In a medium bowl, combine the oat flour, hemp protein, no-calorie sweetener, nutmeg, baking soda, baking powder, and salt and stir to combine.

4. Add the egg whites to the dry ingredients followed by the puréed yogurt/carrot/apple mixture and mix thoroughly.

5. Portion the batter evenly into the muffin cups, filling each about two-thirds full with batter.

6. Bake until a toothpick inserted into the center comes out clean, about 20 minutes. Remove from the oven and allow the muffins to cool on a wire rack. They freeze really well for up to 2 months and will keep in the refrigerator for up to one week.

Per Serving

calories: 123 | fat: 2g | protein: 9g

carbs: 21g | sugars: 6g | fiber: 5g

sodium: 193mg | cholesterol: 1mg

Egg and Vegetable Breakfast Mug

Prep Time: 5 minutes

Cook Time: 2 minutes

Serving: 1

2 eggs

2 tablespoons fat-free milk or plant-based milk

¼ cup thinly sliced spinach

2 cherry tomatoes, halved

2 tablespoons chopped mushroom

4 frozen broccoli florets, chopped

½ teaspoon dried basil

Freshly ground black pepper, to taste

Optional toppings: salsa, sliced avocado, shredded cheese

1. Spray the inside of a large microwave-safe mug, custard cup, or ramekin with cooking spray.

2. Add the eggs and milk to the mug and using a fork, mix until the yolks are combined. Fill the mug two-thirds full (don't fill to the brim), because the eggs will fluff up and expand during the cooking process.

3. Add the spinach, tomatoes, mushroom, broccoli, basil, and pepper to taste. Gently stir to combine.

4. Transfer the mug to the microwave and cook on high for 1 minute.

5. Stir the mixture and microwave for an additional minute or until the eggs are almost set. Cooking times will vary depending on your microwave's strength.

6. Sprinkle with optional toppings, if desired.

Per Serving

calories: 175 | fat: 10g | protein: 15g

carbs: 6g | sugars: 3g | fiber: 1g

sodium: 169mg | cholesterol: 373mg

Greek Yogurt Oat Pancakes

Prep Time: 5 minutes

Prep Time: 5 minutes

Cook Time: 10 minutes

Serving: 2

---

6 egg whites (or ¾ cup liquid egg whites)

1 cup rolled oats

1 cup plain nonfat Greek yogurt

1 medium banana, peeled and sliced

1 teaspoon ground cinnamon

1 teaspoon baking powder

1. In a blender, combine all of the ingredients and blend until smooth. For best results, allow the batter to sit and thicken while the griddle is heating, about 5 minutes.

2. Heat a griddle or large nonstick skillet over medium heat. Spray the skillet with nonstick cooking spray.

3. Pour about one-third cup of the batter onto the griddle. Allow to cook, and flip when bubbles on top burst, about 5 minutes. Cook for another couple of minutes until golden brown. Repeat with the remaining batter.

4. Divide between two serving plates and enjoy.

Per Serving

calories: 318 | fat: 4g | protein: 28g

carbs: 47g | sugars: 13g | fiber: 6g

sodium: 467mg | cholesterol: 5mg

Sweet Potato and Black Bean Hash

Prep Time: 10 minutes

Cook Time: 10 minutes

Serving: 3

1 tablespoon extra-virgin olive oil

1 cup diced peeled sweet potato

1 (15-ounce / 425-g) can black beans, rinsed and drained

1 cup riced cauliflower

4 cherry tomatoes, halved

2 cups baby kale, stems removed, finely chopped, or substitute ⅔ cup frozen

1 teaspoon sweet paprika

Pinch of freshly ground black pepper

1 ounce (about 3 tablespoons / 28 g) unsalted roasted pumpkin seeds

¼ cup chopped fresh cilantro

1. In a medium saucepan, heat the oil over medium-high heat until shimmering, about 30 seconds. Add the sweet potato and cook, stirring frequently until softened and lightly browned, about 5 minutes.

2. Stir in the beans, riced cauliflower, tomatoes, kale, paprika, and black pepper and continue cooking over medium heat until the beans are heated and the kale has wilted, about 5 minutes.

3. Remove from the heat and portion onto 3 plates. Top with the pumpkin seeds and cilantro.

Per Serving

calories: 298 | fat: 10g | protein: 14g

carbs: 42g | sugars: 5g | fiber: 12g

sodium: 45mg | cholesterol: 0mg

Egg in a "Pepper Hole" with Avocado

Prep Time: 15 minutes

Cook Time: 5 minutes

Serving: 4

4 bell peppers, any color

1 tablespoon extra-virgin olive oil

8 large eggs

¾ teaspoon kosher salt, divided

¼ teaspoon freshly ground black pepper, divided

1 avocado, peeled, pitted, and diced

¼ cup red onion, diced

¼ cup fresh basil, chopped

Juice of ½ lime

1. Stem and seed the bell peppers. Cut 2 (2-inch-thick) rings from each pepper. Chop the remaining bell pepper into small dice, and set aside.

2. Heat the olive oil in a large skillet over medium heat. Add 4 bell pepper rings, then crack 1 egg in the middle of each ring. Season with ¼ teaspoon of the salt and ⅛ teaspoon of the black pepper. Cook until the egg whites are mostly set but the yolks are still runny, 2 to 3 minutes. Gently flip and cook 1 additional minute for over easy. Move the egg-bell pepper rings to a platter or onto plates, and repeat with the remaining 4 bell pepper rings.

3. In a medium bowl, combine the avocado, onion, basil, lime juice, reserved diced bell pepper, the remaining ¼ teaspoon kosher salt, and the remaining ⅛ teaspoon black pepper. Divide among the 4 plates.

Per Serving

calories: 270 | fat: 4g | protein: 15g

carbs: 12g | sugars: 6g | fiber: 5g

sodium: 360mg | cholesterol: 370mg

Greek Breakfast Scramble

Prep Time: 10 minutes

Cook Time: 10 minutes

Serving: 4

1 tablespoon olive oil

1 pint grape or cherry tomatoes, quartered

2 cups chopped kale

2 garlic cloves, peeled and minced

8 large eggs

¼ teaspoon kosher or sea salt

¼ teaspoon ground black pepper

¼ cup crumbled feta

¼ cup flat-leaf Italian parsley, chopped

1. Heat the olive oil in a large nonstick skillet over medium heat. Add the tomatoes and kale. Sauté for 2 to 3 minutes, until the kale and tomatoes are slightly soft. Stir in the garlic. Reduce the skillet heat to low.

2. In a medium bowl, whisk together the eggs, salt, and black pepper. Pour the egg mixture into the skillet, slowly folding the eggs until fluffy and scrambled. Remove from the heat and fold in the feta and parsley.

3. Store the scramble in microwaveable airtight containers and refrigerate for up to 5 days. Reheat by microwaving on high for 60 to 90 seconds, until heated through.

Per Serving

calories: 222 | fat: 15g | protein: 15g

carbs: 7g | sugars: 0g | fiber: 1g

sodium: 383mg | cholesterol: 427mg

Strawberry Orange Beet Smoothie

¾ cup unsweetened almond milk

1 tablespoon hemp seeds

1 teaspoon honey

½ teaspoon vanilla extract

½ cup nonfat (0%) plain Greek yogurt

½ cup frozen strawberries

½ navel orange, peeled, quartered, and frozen

½ cup sliced cooked beets (if using canned, use no-salt-added beets)

3 to 4 ice cubes

1. In a high-powered blender, combine the almond milk and hemp seeds and blend on low for 20 to 30 seconds. Add the honey, vanilla, yogurt, strawberries, orange, beets, and ice. Blend until thick and creamy. Serve immediately.

Per Serving

calories: 251 | fat: 6g | protein: 17g

carbs: 32g | sugars: 18g | fiber: 7g

sodium: 239mg | cholesterol: 5mg

Green Apple Pie Protein Smoothie

Prep Time: 5 minutes

Cook Time: 0 minutes

Serving: 1

¾ cup unsweetened vanilla almond or cashew milk

2 tablespoons oat bran

¼ teaspoon apple pie spice or ground cinnamon

½ teaspoon vanilla extract

1 cup baby spinach or ¹/₃ cup frozen

½ cup nonfat (0%) plain Greek yogurt

1 tablespoon avocado

½ medium banana, sliced and frozen

½ cup green apple, unpeeled, chopped and frozen

¼ cup cooked or canned white beans, rinsed and drained

½ cup ice, or to desired consistency

1. In a high-powered blender, combine the milk, oat bran, apple pie spice, vanilla, spinach, yogurt, avocado, banana, apple, beans, and ice. Blend until smooth. Serve immediately.

Per Serving

calories: 319 | fat: 5g | protein: 21g

carbs: 50g | sugars: 19g | fiber: 10g

sodium: 226mg | cholesterol: 5mg

Peach Avocado Smoothie

1½ cups frozen peaches

1½ cups nonfat milk

1 cup nonfat plain or vanilla Greek yogurt

1 avocado, peeled and pitted

1 tablespoon ground flaxseed

1½ teaspoons granulated stevia

1 teaspoon pure vanilla extract

1 to 2 cups ice cubes

Prep Time: 15 minutes

Cook Time: 0 minutes

Serving: 2

1. Combine all the ingredients in a blender. Purée until smooth.

2. Serve immediately.

Per Serving

calories: 323 | fat: 15g | protein: 21g

carbs: 32g | sugars: 21g | fiber: 8g

sodium: 142mg | cholesterol: 9mg

Almond Butter Banana Chocolate Smoothie

¾ cup almond milk

½ medium banana, preferably frozen

¼ cup frozen blueberries

1 tablespoon almond butter

1 tablespoon unsweetened cocoa powder

1 tablespoon chia seeds

Prep Time: 5 minutes

Cook Time: 0 minutes

Serving: 1

1. In a blender or Vitamix, add all the ingredients. Blend to combine.

Per Serving

calories: 300 | fat: 16g | protein: 8g

carbs: 37g | sugars: 17g | fiber: 10g

sodium: 125mg | cholesterol: 0mg

Morning Glory Smoothie

1 cup nonfat milk

½ cup 100% apple juice

2 tablespoons chopped walnuts

2 tablespoons unsweetened coconut flakes

2 frozen bananas

1 small carrot, peeled and chopped

½ teaspoon ground cinnamon

½ teaspoon pure vanilla extract

½ teaspoon granulated stevia

1 to 2 cups ice cubes

1. Place the milk, apple juice, walnuts, and coconut flakes in the pitcher of a blender. Let sit 5 minutes.

2. Add the frozen bananas, carrot, cinnamon, vanilla extract, stevia, and ice cubes to the pitcher. Purée until smooth.

3. Serve immediately.

Per Serving

calories: 276 | fat: 8g | protein: 6g

carbs: 46g | sugars: 30g | fiber: 6g

sodium: 72mg | cholesterol: 2mg

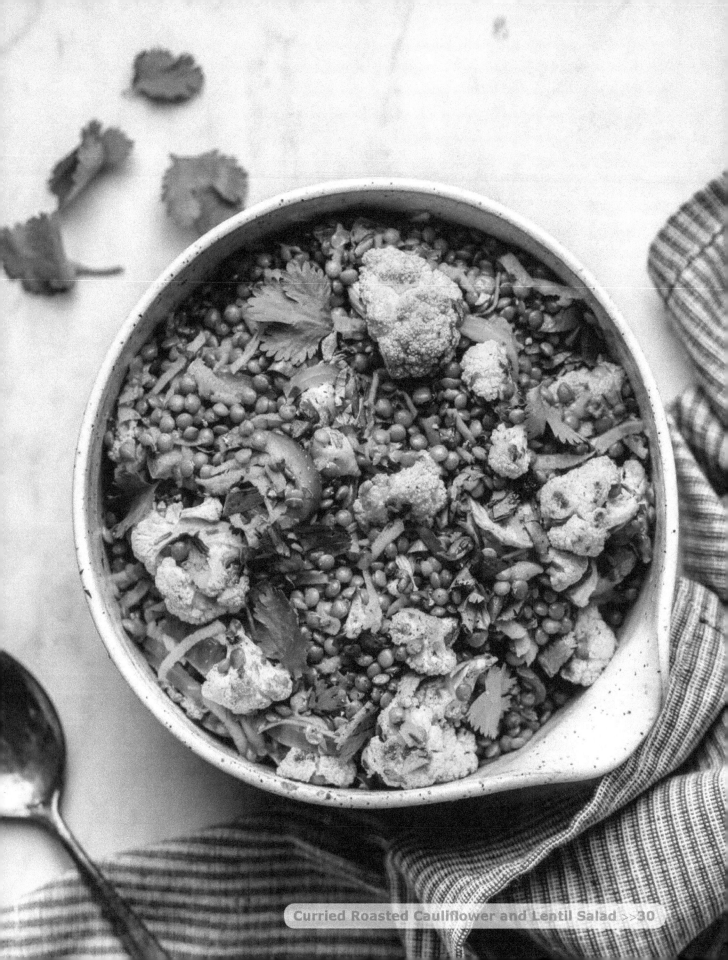

Curried Roasted Cauliflower and Lentil Salad >>30

3 SALADS, SOUPS, AND SANDWICHES

30 Curried Roasted Cauliflower and Lentil Salad

31 Southwestern Chicken Salad

32 Rustic Tomato Panzanella Salad

33 Mediterranean Chickpea Tuna Salad

34 Avocado Egg Salad

35 Roasted Beet, Avocado, and Watercress Salad

36 French Lentil Salad with Parsley

37 Quinoa and Spinach Power Salad

38 Creamy Butternut Squash Soup

39 Quick and Easy Black Bean Soup

40 Creamy Tomato and Greens Soup

41 White Bean Soup with Roasted Eggplant

42 Barley Soup with Asparagus and Mushrooms

43 Two-Potato Cauliflower Soup

44 Chipotle Chicken and Caramelized Onion Panini

45 Spinach and Artichoke Grilled Cheese

46 Black Bean and Beet Burger

Curried Roasted Cauliflower and Lentil Salad

Prep Time: 10 minutes

Cook Time: 25 minutes

Serving: 4

1 head cauliflower, cut into florets

1 small red onion, thinly sliced into half-moons

2 tablespoons extra-virgin olive oil

1 teaspoon ground turmeric

1 teaspoon curry powder

½ teaspoon ground ginger

Pinch of salt

1 cup brown lentils, rinsed

1 bay leaf

¼ cup golden raisins

¾ cup sliced almonds

8 cups mixed baby greens

1 lemon, halved

½ cup loosely packed cilantro leaves

1. Preheat the oven to 400ºF (205ºC). Line a rimmed baking sheet with foil or parchment.

2. In a large bowl, toss the cauliflower florets and sliced onion with the olive oil, turmeric, curry powder, ginger, and salt. Spread in an even layer on the prepared baking sheet. Bake until the cauliflower and onions are tender and lightly browned, about 25 minutes.

3. Meanwhile, in a medium saucepan, combine the lentils and bay leaf and add enough water to cover by 1 inch (about 2 cups). Bring to a boil, reduce the heat, and simmer uncovered until the lentils are tender but not mushy, 16 to 20 minutes.

4. Drain the lentils and discard the bay leaf. Set aside to cool.

5. When everything is cooled, in a medium bowl, toss together the roasted cauliflower and onions, lentils, raisins, and almonds.

6. To assemble the salads, place 2 cups greens on each of 4 serving plates. Divide the cauliflower/lentil mixture among the plates, and top with a squeeze of fresh lemon and the cilantro.

Per Serving

calories: 437 | fat: 20g | protein: 22g
carbs: 53g | sugars: 12g | fiber: 23g
sodium: 141mg | cholesterol: 0mg

Southwestern Chicken Salad

Chicken:

2 boneless, skinless chicken breasts (4 ounces / 113 g each)

1 teaspoon ground cumin

½ teaspoon chili powder

½ teaspoon paprika

Pinch of salt

1 tablespoon extra-virgin olive oil

Salad:

6 cups loosely packed chopped romaine lettuce

1 cup cherry tomatoes, halved

1 cup canned black beans, rinsed and drained

½ cup corn kernels

½ cup shredded low-fat Cheddar cheese

Dressing:

½ avocado

2 tablespoons fresh lime juice

½ cup nonfat (0%) plain Greek yogurt

¼ cup packed fresh cilantro with stems

Pinch of salt

1. Cook the chicken: Season the chicken with cumin, chili powder, paprika, and salt.

2. Heat a large skillet over medium heat and add the olive oil. When shimmering, add the chicken to the pan and cook until it lifts easily with a spatula, 4 to 5 minutes. Flip and continue cooking until a thermometer inserted in the center reads 165ºF (74ºC), another 4 to 5 minutes. Remove from the pan and set aside.

3. Prepare the salad: In a large bowl, toss together the lettuce, tomatoes, beans, corn, and Cheddar. Divide the salad among 4 serving plates.

4. Slice the chicken and divide among the salads.

5. Make the dressing: In a blender or food processor, combine the avocado, lime juice, Greek yogurt, cilantro, and salt and pulse for a few seconds until the cilantro is fully chopped. Top each salad plate with dressing.

Per Serving

calories: 273 | fat: 11g | protein: 24g

carbs: 21g | sugars: 5g | fiber: 7g

sodium: 263mg | cholesterol: 39mg

Rustic Tomato Panzanella Salad

Prep Time: 15 minutes

Cook Time: 8 minutes

Serving: 4

1 small baguette, cubed (about 5 ounces / 142 g total)

3 tablespoons olive oil, divided

2 to 3 large ripe tomatoes, cubed

1 tablespoon red wine vinegar

¼ teaspoon kosher or sea salt

¼ teaspoon ground black pepper

¼ cup fresh basil leaves, torn

1. Preheat the oven to 400ºF (205ºC).

2. Place the cubed baguette on a baking sheet and drizzle with half of the olive oil. Roast in the oven for 8 minutes, until crisp. Transfer the croutons to a mixing bowl.

3. To the bowl, add the tomatoes, red wine vinegar, salt, black pepper, and remaining olive oil. Toss to combine, and top with the fresh basil. Serve immediately.

Per Serving

calories: 200 | fat: 11g | protein: 3g

carbs: 18g | sugars: 0g | fiber: 2g

sodium: 339mg | cholesterol: 0mg

Mediterranean Chickpea Tuna Salad

Prep Time: 20 minutes

Cook Time: 0 minutes

Serving: 4

Dressing:

2 tablespoons red wine vinegar

Zest and juice of ½ lemon

1 tablespoon honey

1 teaspoon dried oregano

leaves

¼ teaspoon kosher or sea salt

¼ teaspoon ground black pepper

¼ cup olive oil

Salad:

1 (15-ounce / 425-g) can no-salt-added chickpeas, rinsed and drained

1 (6.4-ounce / 181-g) pouch albacore tuna

½ English cucumber, diced

1 pint cherry tomatoes, quartered

¼ cup pitted kalamata olives

2 tablespoons crumbled feta cheese

Make the Dressing

1. In a bowl, whisk together red wine vinegar, lemon zest and juice, honey, dried oregano, salt, and black pepper. Slowly whisk in the olive oil until combined.

Make the Salad

2. In a separate bowl, add the chickpeas, tuna, cucumber, tomatoes, olives, and feta cheese.

3. If eating immediately, combine the salad and dressing in a large bowl. If eating later, store the salad and dressing separately in airtight containers. It will stay fresh in the refrigerator for up to 3 days.

Per Serving

calories: 347 | fat: 20g | protein: 17g

carbs: 28g | sugars: 8g | fiber: 6g

sodium: 574mg | cholesterol: 22mg

Avocado Egg Salad

Prep Time: 10 minutes

Cook Time: 20 minutes

Serving: 4

8 large eggs

2 avocados, peeled

Zest and juice of ½ lemon

¼ cup flat-leaf Italian parsley, chopped

¼ teaspoon kosher or sea salt

¼ teaspoon ground black pepper

1. Place the eggs in a saucepan and cover with cold water. Bring to a boil, shut the heat off, and place a fitted lid on the top. Set a timer for 17 to 18 minutes. Drain the hot water, and pour cold water over the eggs until cooled. Remove the shells and discard. Cut the eggs into smaller pieces.

2. In a bowl, mash the avocados. Add the eggs to the bowl, along with the lemon zest and juice, Italian parsley, salt, and ground black pepper. Stir to combine and serve.

Per Serving

calories: 289 | fat: 23g | protein: 14g

carbs: 8g | sugars: 0g | fiber: 6g

sodium: 292mg | cholesterol: 422mg

Roasted Beet, Avocado, and Watercress Salad

Prep Time: 15 minutes

Cook Time: 1 hour

Serving: 4

1 bunch (about 1½ pounds / 680 g) golden beets

1 tablespoon extra-virgin olive oil

1 tablespoon white wine vinegar

½ teaspoon kosher salt

¼ teaspoon freshly ground black pepper

1 bunch (about 4 ounces / 113 g) watercress

1 avocado, peeled, pitted, and diced

¼ cup crumbled feta cheese

¼ cup walnuts, toasted

1 tablespoon fresh chives, chopped

1. Preheat the oven to 425ºF (220ºC). Wash and trim the beets (cut an inch above the beet root, leaving the long tail if desired), then wrap each beet individually in foil. Place the beets on a baking sheet and roast until fully cooked, 45 to 60 minutes depending on the size of each beet. Start checking at 45 minutes; if easily pierced with a fork, the beets are cooked.

2. Remove the beets from the oven and allow them to cool. Under cold running water, slough off the skin. Cut the beets into bite-size cubes or wedges.

3. In a large bowl, whisk together the olive oil, vinegar, salt, and black pepper. Add the watercress and beets and toss well. Add the avocado, feta, walnuts, and chives and mix gently.

Per Serving

calories: 235 | fat: 16g | protein: 6g

carbs: 21g | sugars: 12g | fiber: 8g

sodium: 365mg | cholesterol: 8mg

French Lentil Salad with Parsley

Lentils:

1 cup French lentils

1 garlic clove, smashed

1 dried bay leaf

Salad:

2 tablespoons extra-virgin olive oil

2 tablespoons red wine vinegar

½ teaspoon ground cumin

½ teaspoon kosher salt

¼ teaspoon freshly ground black pepper

2 celery stalks, diced small

1 bell pepper, diced small

½ red onion, diced small

¼ cup fresh parsley, chopped

¼ cup fresh mint, chopped

Make the Lentils

1. Put the lentils, garlic, and bay leaf in a large saucepan. Cover with water by about 3 inches and bring to a boil. Reduce the heat, cover, and simmer until tender, 20 to 30 minutes.

2. Drain the lentils to remove any remaining water after cooking. Remove the garlic and bay leaf.

Make the Salad

3. In a large bowl, whisk together the olive oil, vinegar, cumin, salt, and black pepper. Add the celery, bell pepper, onion, parsley, and mint and toss to combine.

4. Add the lentils and mix well.

Per Serving

calories: 200 | fat: 8g | protein: 10g

carbs: 26g | sugars: 5g | fiber: 10g

sodium: 165mg | cholesterol: 0mg

Quinoa and Spinach Power Salad

½ cup quinoa, rinsed and drained

2 cups spinach, finely chopped

1 medium tomato, diced

1 cup sugar snap peas

½ cup diced cucumbers

¼ cup sliced almonds

½ cup canned chickpeas, rinsed and drained

1½ tablespoons fresh lemon juice

1½ tablespoons extra-virgin olive oil

¼ teaspoon salt

¼ teaspoon freshly ground black pepper

1. In a medium saucepan, combine the quinoa and 1 cup water and bring to a boil over medium-high heat. Reduce the heat to a simmer, cover, and cook until the quinoa has absorbed all of the water, 10 to 15 minutes.

2. Remove from the heat, cover, and let the quinoa steam for 5 minutes. Remove the lid and fluff with a fork.

3. In a large bowl, combine the spinach, tomato, snap peas, cucumbers, almonds, chickpeas, and cooled quinoa.

4. In a small bowl, whisk together the lemon juice, olive oil, salt, and pepper. Pour over the quinoa and vegetables and toss to coat.

5. Portion into 2 serving bowls.

Per Serving

calories: 439 | fat: 20g | protein: 15g

carbs: 54g | sugars: 6g | fiber: 10g

sodium: 333mg | cholesterol: 0mg

Creamy Butternut Squash Soup

Prep Time: 10 minutes

Cook Time: 45 minutes

Serving: 6

1 (12-ounce / 340-g) package cubed peeled butternut squash

1 medium carrot, sliced

1 Granny Smith apple, cubed

1 teaspoon ground cinnamon

½ teaspoon ground ginger

½ teaspoon ground turmeric

½ teaspoon ground nutmeg

2 tablespoons extra-virgin olive oil

1 medium onion, chopped

3 cloves garlic, sliced

4 cups low-sodium vegetable broth

²/₃ cup nonfat (0%) plain Greek yogurt

Salt and freshly ground black pepper, to taste (optional)

1. Preheat the oven to 400ºF (205ºC). Line a rimmed baking sheet with foil.

2. In a medium bowl, combine the butternut squash, carrot, apple, cinnamon, ginger, turmeric, nutmeg, and 1 tablespoon of the olive oil and toss to coat. Spread in an even layer on the baking sheet and roast until softened, 10 to 12 minutes.

3. In a large pot or Dutch oven, heat the remaining 1 tablespoon olive oil over medium-high heat. Add the onion and garlic and cook until tender, 4 to 5 minutes.

4. Add the roasted squash mixture and cook 5 minutes, until heated through, stirring constantly to avoid sticking. Add the broth and simmer for 30 minutes.

5. Remove from the heat and stir in the yogurt. Using an immersion blender, purée the soup until smooth (or transfer in batches to a blender or food processor, purée until smooth, and return to the pot). Stir in salt and pepper, if desired, and simmer gently for 5 minutes.

6. Ladle soup into 6 bowls and serve.

Per Serving

calories: 205 | fat: 7g | protein: 6g

carbs: 32g | sugars: 13g | fiber: 8g

sodium: 178mg | cholesterol: 2mg

Quick and Easy Black Bean Soup

Prep Time: 5 minutes

Cook Time: 15 minutes

Serving: 4

2 (15-ounce / 425-g) cans black beans, rinsed and drained

1 tablespoon extra-virgin olive oil

1 medium onion, diced

4 cloves garlic, minced

2 (14½-ounce / 411-g) cans no-salt-added fire-roasted tomatoes

1 cup low-sodium vegetable broth, plus more as needed

1 teaspoon ground cumin

½ teaspoon chili powder

1 tablespoon fresh lime juice

Salt and freshly ground black pepper, to taste (optional)

½ cup chopped fresh cilantro

1. In a food processor or blender, pulse half of the black beans until thickened but not fully puréed.

2. In a large pot or Dutch oven, heat the olive oil over medium-high heat. Add the onion and garlic and sauté until softened and lightly browned, 4 to 5 minutes.

3. Stir in the processed black beans, the remaining whole black beans, the tomatoes, broth, cumin, and chili powder. Bring to a simmer and cook for 10 to 15 minutes, until thickened. If the soup is too thick, add additional broth; if it is too thin, purée 1 to 2 cups of the soup in a blender and return it to the pot (or use an immersion blender to purée directly in the pot until your desired consistency is reached).

4. Remove from the heat and stir in the lime juice. Season with salt and pepper, if desired. Portion into 4 serving bowls and top with the cilantro.

Per Serving

calories: 262 | fat: 4g | protein: 13g

carbs: 44g | sugars: 9g | fiber: 11g

sodium: 59mg | cholesterol: 0mg

Creamy Tomato and Greens Soup

Prep Time: 5 minutes

Cook Time: 15 minutes

Serving: 4

2 tablespoons extra-virgin olive oil

1 medium red onion, diced

3 cloves garlic, minced

12 Roma (plum) tomatoes, seeded and diced

1 tablespoon tomato paste

1 cup fresh basil leaves

½ teaspoon dried thyme

3 cups low-sodium vegetable broth, plus more as needed

¼ teaspoon freshly ground black pepper

1 cup frozen spinach, thawed

½ cup nonfat (0%) plain Greek yogurt

1. In a large soup pot or Dutch oven, heat the olive oil over medium heat. Add the onion and sauté until translucent, 5 to 7 minutes.

2. Add the garlic and cook for 1 minute. Add the tomatoes, tomato paste, basil, thyme, broth, and black pepper and stir well. Bring the soup to a boil, then reduce the heat and simmer, uncovered, until the tomatoes are very tender, about 30 minutes.

3. Using an immersion blender, purée the soup until smooth (or transfer in batches to a blender or food processor and purée until smooth, returning the soup to the pot).

4. Add the spinach and stir and cook for 4 to 5 minutes, until warmed through.

5. Remove from the heat and allow to cool slightly before stirring in the Greek yogurt (to avoid curdling). This soup has a fairly thick consistency, so if you like a thinner soup, simply add a bit more broth.

Per Serving

calories: 161 | fat: 8g | protein: 7g

carbs: 20g | sugars: 5g | fiber: 6g

sodium: 221mg | cholesterol: 1mg

White Bean Soup with Roasted Eggplant

Prep Time: 20 minutes

Cook Time: 40 minutes

Serving: 4

2 medium red bell peppers, halved

1 medium eggplant, unpeeled, halved lengthwise

1 tablespoon extra-virgin olive oil

1 large onion, chopped

4 cloves garlic, minced

1½ cups low-sodium vegetable broth

2 (15-ounce / 425-g) cans white beans, rinsed and drained

2 teaspoons dried thyme

Salt and freshly ground black pepper, to taste (optional)

Per Serving

calories: 312 | fat: 4g | protein: 15g

carbs: 56g | sugars: 7g | fiber: 14g

sodium: 67mg | cholesterol: 0mg

1. Preheat the broiler. Line a rimmed baking sheet with foil.

2. Place the bell peppers and eggplant halves cut side down on the baking sheet, pressing them down to make them as flat as possible.

3. Broil until the skins are blackened on all sides, 10 to 15 minutes. Remove from the oven and place in a covered container or paper bag or wrap in foil to steam for a few minutes.

4. Meanwhile, in a large pot, heat the olive oil over medium-high heat. Add the onion and garlic and sauté until softened and fragrant, 4 to 5 minutes. Add the broth, beans, and thyme and continue cooking while you peel the eggplant and peppers.

5. When the roasted vegetables are cool enough to handle, scoop the flesh from the eggplant and add to the pot (discard the skin). Remove the charred outer skin from the bell peppers and add the peppers to the pot. Bring the soup to a simmer over medium-low heat and cook for 10 minutes.

6. Using an immersion blender, purée the soup until smooth (or transfer in batches to a blender or food processor and purée until smooth).

7. Taste and add salt and pepper, if desired, and simmer on low for 10 minutes to allow the flavors to develop.

Barley Soup with Asparagus and Mushrooms

Prep Time: 10 minutes

Cook Time: 1 hour

Serving: 4

2 tablespoons extra-virgin olive oil

1 clove garlic, minced

1 medium onion, chopped

1 medium carrot, diced

1 small bunch asparagus, tough ends trimmed, cut into 1- to 2-inch pieces

10 ounces (283 g) mushrooms, sliced

¾ cup pearl barley (or hulled barley, soaked overnight)

4 cups low-sodium vegetable broth

2 bay leaves

1 teaspoon dried marjoram

1 teaspoon sweet paprika

½ teaspoon ground turmeric

1 (15-ounce / 425-g) can white beans, rinsed and drained

4 leaves kale, midribs removed, thinly sliced

3 tablespoons cooking sherry

Freshly ground black pepper, to taste (optional)

¼ cup minced fresh parsley

1. In a large soup pot, heat the olive oil over medium heat. Add the garlic, onion, and carrot and cook, stirring occasionally, until the vegetables have softened, 8 to 10 minutes.

2. Add the asparagus and mushrooms, stir well, and continue to cook for another 5 minutes.

3. Add the barley, broth, bay leaves, marjoram, paprika, and turmeric and bring to a boil. Reduce the heat to low, cover, and simmer until the barley is tender and plumps up, 30 to 40 minutes for pearl barley, 60 minutes for hulled barley. If the soup seems too thick at any point, add more water, ½ cup at a time.

4. When the barley is tender, stir in the beans, kale, and sherry and continue to cook for 10 minutes.

5. Season with pepper, if desired, and stir in the parsley before serving.

Per Serving

calories: 372 | fat: 8g | protein: 14g

carbs: 69g | sugars: 7g | fiber: 15g

sodium: 173mg | cholesterol: 0mg

Two-Potato Cauliflower Soup

Prep Time: 15 minutes

Cook Time: 30 minutes

Serving: 4

---

1 tablespoon extra-virgin olive oil

1 leek, thinly sliced

2 cloves garlic, minced

2 cups cauliflower florets

½ pound (227 g) sweet potatoes, peeled and chopped

½ pound (227 g) Yukon Gold potatoes, unpeeled and chopped

3 cups low-sodium vegetable broth

1 cup fat-free milk or plant-based milk

1 teaspoon sweet paprika

½ teaspoon freshly ground black pepper, or more to taste

¼ cup chopped fresh chives (optional)

1. In a large soup pot or saucepan, heat the olive oil over medium heat. Add the leek and cook until softened, 3 to 5 minutes. Add the garlic and cook for 1 minute.

2. Stir in the cauliflower, sweet potatoes, gold potatoes, and broth and bring to a boil. Reduce the heat, cover, and simmer until the vegetables are tender, 15 to 20 minutes.

3. Using an immersion blender, purée the soup until smooth (or transfer in batches to a blender or food processor and purée until smooth, then return to the pot).

4. Stir in the milk, paprika, and black pepper and cook for 3 to 5 minutes more to heat through.

5. Serve topped with fresh chives, if desired.

Per Serving

calories: 181 | fat: 4g | protein: 6g

carbs: 33g | sugars: 10g | fiber: 6g

sodium: 182mg | cholesterol: 1mg

Chipotle Chicken and Caramelized Onion Panini

Prep Time: 20 minutes

Cook Time: 25 minutes

Serving: 8

2 tablespoons canola oil, divided

2 yellow onions, thinly sliced

½ pound (227 g) boneless skinless chicken breasts, thinly sliced

2 tablespoons Honey Chipotle Sauce (see recipe)

8 slices store-bought whole-wheat bread

4 slices low-sodium provolone cheese

1 tablespoon olive oil

Per Serving

calories: 260 | fat: 11g | protein: 20g

carbs: 25g | sugars: 7g | fiber: 3g

sodium: 308mg | cholesterol: 26mg

1. In a large skillet, heat 2 tablespoons canola oil over medium-low heat. Add the onions and cook for 20 minutes, stirring occasionally, until they are soft and caramel colored on the edges. Place them in a bowl and set aside.

2. In the same skillet, add another tablespoon of canola oil over medium heat. Place the chicken in the skillet and cook for 3 to 4 minutes per side, until the chicken reaches 165ºF (74ºC). Transfer the cooked chicken to the bowl with the caramelized onions and stir in the honey chipotle sauce until combined.

3. Wipe out the skillet and put back on the range. Prepare the sandwiches by placing 4 slices of bread on a cutting board. Evenly distribute the chicken/onion mixture onto each slice and top with a slice of provolone cheese. Top with another slice of bread. Brush the top slices of bread with olive oil. Place the sandwiches olive oil-side down in the hot skillet. Cook for 2 to 3 minutes, until browned. Brush the other slices of bread with olive oil, then flip and cook for another 2 to 3 minutes, until the bottom is browned and the cheese is melted. Place a lid over the skillet, if necessary, to assist with melting the cheese.

4. Slice each sandwich in half and serve.

Spinach and Artichoke Grilled Cheese

Prep Time: 15 minutes

Cook Time: 15 minutes

Serving: 4

2 cups baby spinach leaves, chopped

1 cup jarred marinated artichoke hearts, chopped

¼ cup nonfat plain Greek yogurt

2 to 3 garlic cloves, peeled and minced

¼ teaspoon ground black pepper

⅛ teaspoon kosher or sea salt

8 slices whole-wheat bread

4 slices Mozzarella cheese

1 tablespoon olive oil

1. In a bowl, mix together the spinach, artichoke hearts, Greek yogurt, garlic, black pepper, and salt until combined.

2. Heat a skillet to medium. Prepare the sandwiches by placing 4 slices bread on a cutting board. Evenly distribute the spinach artichoke mixture onto each slice and top with a slice of Mozzarella cheese. Top with another slice of bread. Brush top slices of bread with the olive oil. Place the sandwiches olive oil-side down in the hot skillet. Cook for 2 to 3 minutes, until browned. Brush the other slices of bread with the olive oil, then flip and cook for another 2 to 3 minutes, until the bottom is browned and the cheese is melted. Place a lid over the skillet, if necessary, to assist with melting the cheese.

3. Slice each sandwich in half and serve.

Per Serving

calories: 355 | fat: 13g | protein: 16g

carbs: 44g | sugars: 7g | fiber: 9g

sodium: 511mg | cholesterol: 11mg

Black Bean and Beet Burger

Prep Time: 20 minutes

Cook Time: 30 minutes

Serving: 6

1 tablespoon chia seeds

1 (15-ounce / 425-g) can black beans, rinsed and drained

¼ pound (113 g) cooked and peeled beets, quartered (2 medium)

½ cup steel-cut oats

1 cup sliced mushrooms

1 teaspoon dry mustard

1 teaspoon ground cumin

½ teaspoon smoked paprika

1 teaspoon Bragg liquid aminos or reduced-sodium soy sauce

1 teaspoon vegan Worcestershire sauce

1 teaspoon minced garlic

Pinch of salt

2 tablespoons chickpea flour or other whole-grain flour, plus more as needed

Lettuce leaves or whole-grain buns

Per Serving

calories: 132 | fat: 1g | protein: 7g

carbs: 24g | sugars: 2g | fiber: 6g

sodium: 89mg | cholesterol: 0mg

1. In a small bowl, combine the chia seeds and 3 tablespoons water to make a chia "egg." Set aside for 5 minutes, until the mixture forms a gel.

2. Meanwhile, in a medium bowl, coarsely mash ½ cup of the black beans with a fork, leaving some texture.

3. In a food processor, combine the remaining black beans, the chia "egg," beets, oats, mushrooms, mustard, cumin, paprika, liquid aminos, Worcestershire sauce, garlic, and salt. Pulse until the ingredients are combined but not completely pulverized. You want the burgers to have some texture.

4. Add the contents of the food processor to the bowl with the mashed beans. Add the chickpea flour and mix (it might be easier to use your hands) until the ingredients hold together, adding more flour as needed. Refrigerate to chill for 10 minutes while you preheat the oven. Chilling helps the burgers hold together better.

5. Preheat the oven to 375ºF (190ºC). Coat a baking sheet with cooking spray.

6. Remove the mixture from the fridge and form it into 6 evenly sized balls, then use the palm of your hand to gently flatten into patties.

7. Arrange the burgers on the baking sheet and lightly spray the tops with cooking spray. Bake for 30 minutes to heat through, until lightly browned, gently turning halfway through cooking.

8. Serve on lettuce leaves or toasted whole-grain buns.

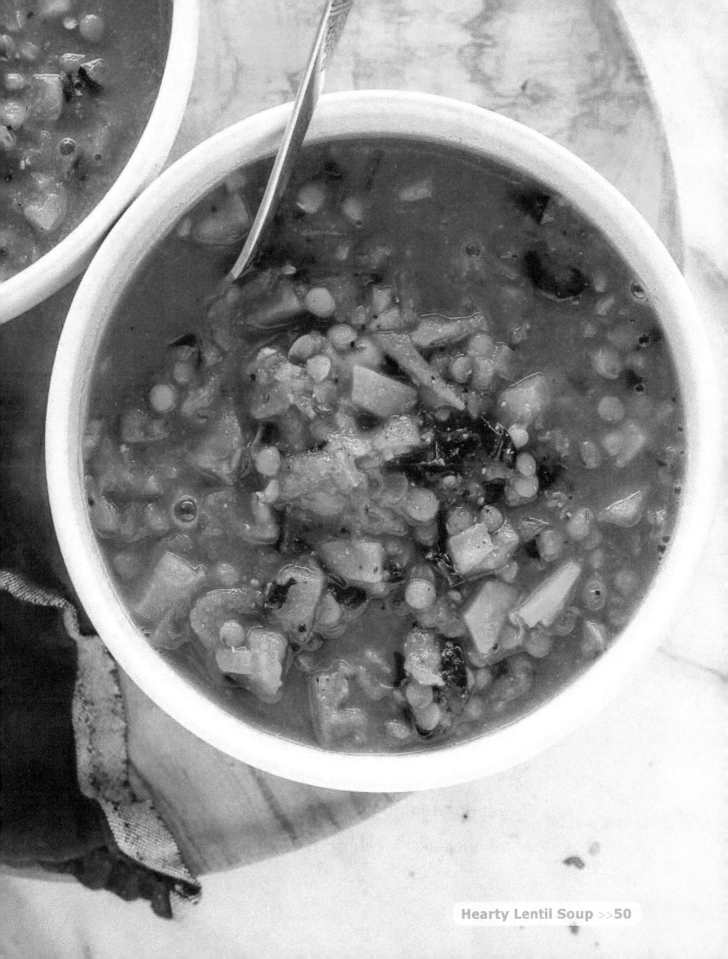

4 VEGETARIAN AND VEGAN MAINS

49 Southwest Tofu Scramble

50 Hearty Lentil Soup

51 Loaded Baked Sweet Potatoes

52 White Beans with Spinach and Tomatoes

53 Coconut Rice and White Beans

54 Cauliflower Butternut Squash Mac and Cheese

55 Bean Pasta with Arugula Avocado Walnut Pesto

56 Lentil Sloppy Joes

57 Lentil-Walnut Mushroom Tacos

58 Cauliflower "Fried Rice" and Mixed Vegetables

59 Mushroom and Sweet Potato Mini Quiches

60 Almond Butter Tofu and Roasted Asparagus

61 Spicy Bean Chili

62 Herbed Mushroom Rice

63 Pasta Primavera

64 Penne with White Beans and Tomatoes

65 Sweet Potato and Black Bean Wraps

66 Asparagus and Mushroom Crustless Quiche

Southwest Tofu Scramble

Prep Time: 10 minutes

Cook Time: 15 minutes

Serving: 1

½ tablespoon olive oil

½ red onion, chopped

2 cups chopped spinach

8 ounces (227 g) firm tofu, drained well

1 teaspoon ground cumin

½ teaspoon garlic powder

Optional for serving: sliced avocado or sliced tomatoes

1. Heat the olive oil in a medium skillet over medium heat. Add the onion and cook until softened, about 5 minutes.

2. Add the spinach and cover to steam for 2 minutes.

3. Using a spatula, move the veggies to one side of the pan. Crumble the tofu into the open area in the pan, breaking it up with a fork. Add the cumin and garlic to the crumbled tofu and mix well. Sauté for 5 to 7 minutes until the tofu is slightly browned.

4. Serve immediately with whole-grain bread, fruit, or beans. Top with optional sliced avocado and tomato, if using.

Per Serving

calories: 267 | fat: 17g | protein: 23g

carbs: 13g | sugars: 2g | fiber: 5g

sodium: 75mg | cholesterol: 0mg

Hearty Lentil Soup

Prep Time: 10 minutes

Cook Time: 30 minutes

Serving: 4

1 tablespoon olive oil

2 carrots, peeled and chopped

2 celery stalks, diced

1 onion, chopped

1 teaspoon dried thyme

½ teaspoon garlic powder

Freshly ground black pepper, to taste

1 (28-ounce / 794-g) can no-salt diced tomatoes, drained

1 cup dry lentils

5 cups water

Salt, to taste

1. Heat the oil in a large Dutch oven or pot over medium heat. Once the oil is simmering, add the carrot, celery, and onion. Cook, stirring often, until the onion has softened and is turning translucent, about 5 minutes. Add the thyme, garlic powder, and black pepper. Cook until fragrant while stirring constantly, about 30 seconds.

2. Pour in the drained diced tomatoes and cook for a few more minutes, stirring often, in order to enhance their flavor.

3. Add the lentils, water, and a pinch of salt. Raise the heat and bring to a boil, then partially cover the pot and reduce heat to maintain a gentle simmer. Cook for 30 minutes, or until lentils are tender but still hold their shape.

4. Ladle into serving bowls and serve with a fresh green salad and whole-grain bread.

Per Serving

calories: 168 | fat: 4g | protein: 10g

carbs: 35g | sugars: 8g | fiber: 14g

sodium: 130mg | cholesterol: 0mg

Loaded Baked Sweet Potatoes

Prep Time: 10 minutes

Cook Time: 20 minutes

Serving: 4

4 sweet potatoes

½ cup nonfat or low-fat plain Greek yogurt

Freshly ground black pepper, to taste

1 teaspoon olive oil

1 red bell pepper, cored and diced

½ red onion, diced

1 teaspoon ground cumin

1 (15-ounce / 425-g) can chickpeas, drained and rinsed

1. Poke holes in the potatoes with a fork and cook on your microwave's potato setting until potatoes are soft and cooked through, about 8 to 10 minutes for 4 potatoes. If you don't have a microwave, bake at 400ºF (205ºC) for about 45 minutes.

2. Combine the yogurt and black pepper in a small bowl and mix well.

3. Heat the oil in a medium pot over medium heat. Add bell pepper, onion, cumin, and additional black pepper to taste.

4. Add the chickpeas, stir to combine, and heat through, about 5 minutes.

5. Slice the potatoes lengthwise down the middle and top each half with a portion of the bean mixture followed by 1 to 2 tablespoons of the yogurt.

6. Serve immediately.

Per Serving

calories: 364 | fat: 2g | protein: 11g

carbs: 51g | sugars: 1g | fiber: 10g

sodium: 124mg | cholesterol: 1mg

White Beans with Spinach and Tomatoes

Prep Time: 15 minutes

Cook Time: 10 minutes

Serving: 2

1 tablespoon olive oil

4 small plum tomatoes, halved lengthwise

10 ounces (283 g) frozen spinach, defrosted and squeezed of excess water

2 garlic cloves, thinly sliced

2 tablespoons water

¼ teaspoon freshly ground black pepper

1 (15-ounce / 425-g) can white beans, drained and rinsed

Juice of 1 lemon

1. Heat the oil in a large skillet over medium-high heat. Add the tomatoes, cut-side down, and cook, shaking the pan occasionally, until browned and starting to soften, 3 to 5 minutes; turn and cook for 1 minute more. Transfer to a plate.

2. Reduce heat to medium and add the spinach, garlic, water, and pepper to the skillet. Cook, tossing, until the spinach is heated through, 2 to 3 minutes.

3. Return the tomatoes to the skillet, add the white beans and lemon juice, and toss until heated through, 1 to 2 minutes.

Per Serving

calories: 293 | fat: 9g | protein: 15g

carbs: 43g | sugars: 1g | fiber: 16g

sodium: 267mg | cholesterol: 0mg

Coconut Rice and White Beans

Prep Time: 10 minutes

Cook Time: 30 minutes

Serving: 2

1 stalk lemongrass, bottom 6 inches only, outer leaves peeled

1 teaspoon extra-virgin olive oil

2 cloves garlic, minced

2 tablespoons minced shallot

½ cup chopped red bell pepper

1 cup cubed and peeled eggplant

1 teaspoon ground cardamom

1 teaspoon ground coriander

½ teaspoon ground cinnamon

½ cup canned no-salt-added diced tomatoes and their juices

½ cup black rice

⅔ cup canned "lite" coconut milk

1 (15-ounce / 425-g) can small white beans, rinsed and drained

2 cups chopped baby kale

½ lime

Hot sauce (optional)

Salt and freshly ground black pepper, to taste (optional)

1. Lightly pound the lemongrass stalk with a kitchen mallet.

2. In a large pot, heat the olive oil over high heat. Add the garlic and shallot and cook until soft, 3 to 5 minutes. Add the bell pepper and eggplant and continue cooking until softened, 3 to 5 minutes.

3. Add the cardamom, coriander, and cinnamon and cook for 1 more minute, stirring occasionally to prevent the spices from burning.

4. Add the tomatoes, black rice, coconut milk, 1½ cups water, and beans and stir to combine. Cover, bring to a boil, then reduce the heat to low and allow to simmer for 20 minutes.

5. Stir in the kale, cover, and continue cooking until the kale is wilted, the rice is done, and most of the liquid is absorbed, 5 to 8 minutes longer.

6. To serve, remove the lemongrass stalk and squeeze in the lime juice. If desired, season with hot sauce and a dash of salt and black pepper.

Per Serving

calories: 433 | fat: 9g | protein: 19g

carbs: 75g | sugars: 6g | fiber: 16g

sodium: 32mg | cholesterol: 0mg

Cauliflower Butternut Squash Mac and Cheese

Prep Time: 10 minutes

Cook Time: 20 minutes

Serving: 4

---

8 ounces (227 g) chickpea pasta elbows

2 cups cubed peeled butternut squash

2 cups cauliflower florets

2 cups fat-free milk

½ teaspoon freshly ground black pepper

Dash of salt

½ tablespoon extra-virgin olive oil

½ medium red onion, minced

2 cloves garlic, minced

2 teaspoons Dijon mustard

2 teaspoons sweet paprika

1 cup shredded low-fat Cheddar cheese

½ cup part-skim ricotta cheese

1. Cook the pasta according to the package directions. Drain and set aside.

2. In a medium saucepan, combine the butternut squash, cauliflower, and 1 cup of the milk. Season with the pepper and salt. Bring to a simmer over medium-high heat, then reduce the heat to low, cover, and cook until fork-tender, 8 to 10 minutes. Transfer the cooked vegetables to a food processor or blender and purée until smooth.

3. Meanwhile, in a large saucepan, heat the olive oil over medium-high heat. Add the onion and garlic and sauté until tender, 3 to 5 minutes.

4. Add the vegetable purée, the remaining 1 cup milk, the mustard, and paprika to the saucepan and bring to a simmer. Cook until starting to thicken, about 5 minutes.

5. Add the Cheddar and ricotta cheese and stir to combine. Add the drained pasta to the pan and stir to combine.

6. Serve immediately.

Per Serving

calories: 372 | fat: 9g | protein: 28g

carbs: 53g | sugars: 13g | fiber: 13g

sodium: 405mg | cholesterol: 15mg

Bean Pasta with Arugula Avocado Walnut Pesto

Prep Time: 10 minutes

Cook Time: 5 minutes

Serving: 4

2 cups packed arugula

1 cup packed fresh basil leaves

¼ cup chopped walnuts

²/₃ cup green peas (thawed if frozen)

½ medium avocado

3 cloves garlic, coarsely chopped

2 tablespoons fresh lemon juice

¼ cup nutritional yeast

Pinch of salt

3 tablespoons extra-virgin olive oil

8 ounces (227 g) bean pasta

Fresh parsley (optional)

1. Fill a large saucepan three-quarters full with water and bring to a rolling boil over high heat.

2. Meanwhile, in a food processor, combine the arugula, basil, walnuts, peas, avocado, garlic, lemon juice, nutritional yeast, and salt and pulse until finely chopped. Add the olive oil and continue to process the pesto until creamy or the desired consistency is reached.

3. Add the pasta to the boiling water and cook to al dente, according to the package directions, being certain not to overcook. Drain the pasta and transfer to a bowl. Add the pesto and toss to combine.

4. Portion onto 4 serving plates and garnish with fresh parsley, if desired.

Per Serving

calories: 417 | fat: 22g | protein: 21g

carbs: 43g | sugars: 7g | fiber: 13g

sodium: 122mg | cholesterol: 0mg

Lentil Sloppy Joes

Prep Time: 15 minutes

Cook Time: 20 minutes

Serving: 4

1 cup green or brown lentils, rinsed

¼ cup unsweetened dried apricots, chopped

2 tablespoons tomato paste

½ teaspoon yellow mustard

½ tablespoon extra-virgin olive oil

½ medium yellow onion, diced

1 medium green bell pepper, diced

1 large stalk celery, diced

½ cup grated carrot

3 cloves garlic, minced

1 (15-ounce / 425-g) can tomato sauce

1 tablespoon red wine vinegar

1 tablespoon vegetarian Worcestershire sauce

2 teaspoons chili powder

1 teaspoon ground cumin

1 teaspoon smoked or sweet paprika

Lettuce leaves or whole-grain buns

1. In a small saucepan, combine the lentils and 2 cups water. Bring to a boil, reduce the heat, and simmer, covered, until tender but not falling apart, 20 to 25 minutes. Drain and set aside.

2. Meanwhile, in a food processor or blender, combine the dried apricots, tomato paste, and mustard and process/blend until the apricots are blended into a paste. Transfer the apricot paste to a small bowl and set aside.

3. Heat a large skillet over medium-high heat. Add the olive oil, onion, bell pepper, celery, carrot, and garlic and stir to combine. Cook, stirring frequently, until the vegetables are slightly browned and tender, 4 to 5 minutes.

4. Add the apricot paste, tomato sauce, vinegar, Worcestershire sauce, chili powder, cumin, and paprika to the skillet. Stir to combine and cook until the spices are fragrant, 2 minutes.

5. Add the drained lentils to the pan and stir well to combine. Continue cooking over medium-low heat until the sauce thickens, stirring occasionally, 5 to 10 minutes. Taste and adjust seasonings before serving.

6. Ladle the mixture onto lettuce leaves or toasted buns.

Per Serving

calories: 269 | fat: 3g | protein: 15g

carbs: 50g | sugars: 13g | fiber: 17g

sodium: 559mg | cholesterol: 0mg

Lentil-Walnut Mushroom Tacos

Prep Time: 20 minutes

Cook Time: 30 minutes

Serving: 5

¼ cup green or brown lentils, rinsed

4 portobello mushrooms

¼ cup unsalted pistachios

¼ cup walnut halves

2 tablespoons chopped canned chipotle peppers in adobo sauce

2 cups riced cauliflower

1 teaspoon chili powder

1 teaspoon ground coriander

1 teaspoon ground cumin

1 teaspoon garlic powder

1 teaspoon dried oregano

1 teaspoon smoked paprika

Juice of 1 lime

Per Serving

calories: 346 | fat: 19g | protein: 19g

carbs: 33g | sugars: 16g | fiber: 15g

sodium: 141mg | cholesterol: 0mg

1. In a small saucepan, cook the lentils in water to cover over medium-high heat until tender, 20 to 25 minutes. Drain and set aside.

2. Meanwhile, preheat the oven to 375ºF (190ºC). Line a large baking sheet with parchment paper.

3. Remove the stems and carefully scrape out the gills from the mushrooms using a small paring knife. Transfer to a food processor.

4. In a dry medium skillet, toast the pistachios and walnuts, stirring constantly, until lightly golden, 2 to 3 minutes.

5. Scrape the nuts into the food processor. Add the chipotle peppers in adobo sauce and the drained lentils. Pulse lightly until the ingredients are combined, being careful not to overprocess as you want there to be some texture.

6. In a medium bowl, combine the riced cauliflower, chili powder, coriander cumin, garlic powder, oregano, and paprika. Add the contents of the food processor to the bowl and mix until everything is combined.

7. Spread the mixture on the parchment and drizzle with lime juice. Bake for 15 minutes. Use a spatula to turn the mixture, and also make room for the portobello mushroom caps. Coat both sides of the caps lightly with cooking spray. Return to the oven and bake until the mushroom caps are lightly browned and the lentil mixture is lightly browned and crumbly but not overly dry, 15 minutes to 20 minutes longer.

8. Remove the pan from the oven and give the lentil mixture a good stir.

9. To serve, place 2 mushroom caps on each of 2 serving plates and top with the lentil-nut "meat."

Cauliflower "Fried Rice" and Mixed Vegetables

Prep Time: 10 minutes

Cook Time: 15 minutes

Serving: 4

1 tablespoon plus 1 teaspoon sesame oil

1 cup chopped scallions, white and green parts separated

2 cloves garlic, minced

1 teaspoon grated fresh ginger

1 red bell pepper, chopped

1 cup frozen shelled edamame, thawed

1 cup mushrooms, sliced

4 cups fresh or frozen riced cauliflower

2 egg whites, whisked

1 large egg, beaten

1 tablespoon reduced-sodium soy sauce

1 tablespoon balsamic vinegar

Pinch of red pepper flakes

¼ cup chopped peanuts or cashews

1. In a large wok or nonstick skillet, heat 1 tablespoon of the sesame oil over medium-high heat. Add the scallion whites, garlic, and ginger and cook, stirring often, until fragrant but not browned, 2 to 3 minutes.

2. Add the bell pepper, edamame, and mushrooms and cook until the pepper is softened, about 2 minutes. Add the cauliflower rice, stir to combine, and stir-fry quickly to cook the cauliflower to a soft but not mushy texture, 5 to 7 minutes.

3. Make a well in the center of the vegetables. Reduce the heat, add the remaining 1 teaspoon sesame oil to the center, and add the egg whites and whole egg. Stir gently and constantly until the eggs are fully cooked, then stir together with the cauliflower rice.

4. Stir in the scallion greens, the soy sauce, balsamic vinegar, and pepper flakes and cook for 1 minute.

5. Serve garnished with chopped nuts.

Per Serving

calories: 219 | fat: 12g | protein: 15g

carbs: 17g | sugars: 4g | fiber: 6g

sodium: 219mg | cholesterol: 46mg

Mushroom and Sweet Potato Mini Quiches

Prep Time: 5 minutes

Cook Time: 35 minutes

Serving: 2

1 cup chickpea flour

¼ cup nutritional yeast

1 teaspoon baking powder

2 teaspoons ground sage

1 teaspoon dried thyme

1 teaspoon ground turmeric

Pinch of salt (black salt, if possible)

Freshly ground black pepper, to taste

1 cup unsweetened cashew milk (or fat-free dairy milk if you are not vegan)

$^2/_3$ cup frozen green peas, slightly thawed

1 cup riced cauliflower and sweet potato

1 cup finely chopped button mushrooms

1 teaspoon minced garlic

1 tablespoon minced shallot

1. Preheat the oven to 375ºF (190ºC). For a main course, lightly coat four 1-cup ramekins with cooking spray; for a snack or side, spray 8 cups of a muffin tin.

2. In a medium bowl, stir together the chickpea flour, nutritional yeast, baking powder, sage, thyme, turmeric, salt, and black pepper to taste. Stir in the milk.

3. Add the peas, riced cauliflower and sweet potato, mushrooms, garlic, and shallot and mix to combine. The batter will be thin.

4. Divide the batter evenly among the prepared ramekins or muffin cups. Transfer to the oven and bake until firm to the touch and lightly browned, about 35 minutes.

5. Remove from the oven and let sit for an additional 10 minutes (they will continue to firm up), then transfer to a wire rack and allow to cool slightly if eating immediately or completely if storing for later. Store in an airtight container in the refrigerator for up to 1 week.

Per Serving

calories: 356 | fat: 1g | protein: 23g

carbs: 57g | sugars: 11g | fiber: 16g

sodium: 178mg | cholesterol: 0mg

Almond Butter Tofu and Roasted Asparagus

Prep Time: 15 minutes

Cook Time: 40 minutes

Serving: 3

1 (14-ounce / 397-g) block extra-firm tofu

1 tablespoon sesame oil

1 tablespoon pure maple syrup

2 tablespoons reduced-sodium tamari

2 tablespoons almond butter

2 tablespoons fresh lime juice

1 tablespoon balsamic vinegar

3 cloves garlic, minced

1 pound (454 g) asparagus, tough ends trimmed

1 tablespoon extra-virgin olive oil

Freshly ground black pepper, to taste (optional)

Chili hot sauce (e.g. Sriracha) (optional)

Per Serving

calories: 337 | fat: 21g | protein: 21g

carbs: 21g | sugars: 8g | fiber: 6g

sodium: 496mg | cholesterol: 0mg

1. Pat tofu dry and roll in a clean absorbent towel and place something heavy on top such as a heavy skillet or plates with a can on top, for at least 15 minutes (up to 1 hour) in order to remove excess water.

2. Preheat the oven to 400°F (205°C). Coat two large baking sheets with cooking spray.

3. Unwrap the tofu and cut into 1-inch cubes. Arrange on one of the prepared baking sheets in an even layer and bake until puffy and slightly browned, 20 to 25 minutes.

4. Meanwhile, in a small bowl, combine the sesame oil, maple syrup, tamari, almond butter, lime juice, balsamic vinegar, and two-thirds of the minced garlic. Whisk to combine. Set the marinade aside.

5. In a medium bowl, drizzle the asparagus with the olive oil, then toss to coat. Sprinkle with the remaining garlic and season with black pepper, if desired. Arrange the asparagus in a single layer on the second baking sheet.

6. Remove the tofu from the oven and place the asparagus in the oven in its place. Add the baked tofu to the marinade and toss to coat. Let marinate for 5 minutes, stirring occasionally.

7. Heat a large skillet over medium heat. Once hot, add the tofu (reserve the marinade) and cook, stirring occasionally, until browned on all sides, about 5 minutes.

8. Remove the roasted asparagus from the oven and add to the skillet with the tofu along with the reserved marinade. Cook for an additional 2 minutes, stirring frequently.

9. Garnish with hot sauce, if desired.

Spicy Bean Chili

Prep Time: 15 minutes

Cook Time: 20 minutes

Serving: 4

---

2 teaspoons olive oil

1 medium red onion, thinly sliced

2 garlic cloves, minced

2 (15-ounce / 425-g) cans kidney beans, drained and rinsed

1 (8-ounce / 227-g) can no-salt crushed tomatoes

1 cup low-sodium vegetable broth

½ cup water

2 teaspoons chili powder

¼ teaspoon ground cinnamon

1. Heat the olive oil in a large saucepan over medium-high heat. Add the onion and sauté until the onion is lightly caramelized, about 5 minutes. Add the garlic and sauté until fragrant, about 30 seconds.

2. Stir in the remaining ingredients and bring to a boil on high for 1 minute. Cover, reduce heat to low, and simmer until flavors are well combined, about 10 minutes.

3. Enjoy immediately.

Per Serving

calories: 223 | fat: 4g | protein: 12g

carbs: 37g | sugars: 1g | fiber: 13g

sodium: 237mg | cholesterol: 0mg

Herbed Mushroom Rice

2 teaspoons olive oil

12 ounces (340 g) sliced mushrooms

3 scallion stalks, thinly sliced and separated

¾ teaspoon freshly ground black pepper

2 cups water

1 teaspoon dried rosemary

1 cup dry instant brown rice

2 cups frozen lima beans

¼ cup shredded Romano cheese (optional)

1. Heat the olive oil in a large saucepan over medium-high heat. Add the mushrooms, the white parts of the scallions, and the black pepper and sauté until the mushrooms are just cooked through, about 5 minutes.

2. Add the water and rosemary, and bring to a boil over high heat. Stir in the rice, lima beans, and half of the green parts of the scallions, and reduce the heat to medium. Cook, stirring occasionally, for 6 to 8 minutes, or until the rice is cooked and the lima beans are tender.

3. Sprinkle each serving with cheese (if using) and the remaining green parts of the scallions. Serve immediately.

Per Serving

calories: 220 | fat: 4g | protein: 10g

carbs: 40g | sugars: 1g | fiber: 9g

sodium: 11mg | cholesterol: 0mg

Pasta Primavera

Prep Time: 10 minutes

Cook Time: 15 minutes

Serving: 4

---

2 cups broccoli florets

1 cup sliced mushrooms

1 cup sliced zucchini or yellow squash

1 tablespoon olive oil, plus 1 teaspoon

2 garlic cloves, minced

¾ cup fat-free evaporated milk

½ cup freshly grated Parmesan cheese

8 ounces (227 g) whole-wheat angel-hair or spaghetti pasta

1/3 cup chopped fresh parsley (optional)

Per Serving

calories: 350 | fat: 9g | protein: 17g

carbs: 53g | sugars: 7g | fiber: 7g

sodium: 317mg | cholesterol: 12mg

1. In a large pot fitted with a steamer basket, bring about 1 inch of water to a boil. Add the broccoli, mushrooms, and zucchini. Cover and steam until tender-crisp, about 10 minutes. Remove from the pot.

2. In a large saucepan, heat 1 tablespoon of the olive oil over medium heat. Add the garlic and sauté over medium heat for 2 to 3 minutes. Add the steamed vegetables and stir or shake to coat the vegetables with the garlic. Remove the saucepan from the heat but keep warm.

3. In another large saucepan, heat the remaining 1 teaspoon of olive oil, evaporated milk, and Parmesan cheese. Stir continuously over medium heat until somewhat thickened and heated through without scalding. Remove the saucepan from the heat but keep warm.

4. Fill a large pot three-quarters full with water and bring to a boil. Add the pasta and cook according to the package directions, until the desired doneness. Drain the pasta.

5. Divide the pasta evenly among four plates. Top each serving with a quarter of the vegetables and Parmesan sauce. Garnish with fresh parsley (if using) and serve immediately.

Penne with White Beans and Tomatoes

Prep Time: 5 minutes

Cook Time: 25 minutes

Serving: 4

---

2 pints cherry tomatoes, halved

2 tablespoons chopped fresh basil

2 tablespoons olive oil, divided

8 ounces (227 g) whole-wheat penne

2 garlic cloves, minced

1 (15-ounce / 425-g) can white beans (navy or great northern), drained and rinsed

1 tablespoon balsamic vinegar

1. Preheat the oven to 425ºF (220ºC).

2. On a large sheet pan, toss the tomatoes with the basil and 1 tablespoon of the olive oil. Place the pan in the oven and roast until wilted and beginning to brown, about 20 minutes.

3. Meanwhile, cook the penne according to the package directions. Reserve ¼ cup of the cooking water, and drain. Add the pasta, beans, tomato mixture, garlic, balsamic vinegar, and the cooking water to a medium pot and simmer for 2 minutes.

4. Drizzle the pasta with the remaining 1 tablespoon of olive oil and serve.

Per Serving

calories: 370 | fat: 9g | protein: 13g

carbs: 66g | sugars: 1g | fiber: 6g

sodium: 121mg | cholesterol: 0mg

Sweet Potato and Black Bean Wraps

Prep Time: 10 minutes

Cook Time: 20 minutes

Serving: 4

---

1 large sweet potato, cubed

2 teaspoons olive oil

½ small onion, finely chopped

1 bell pepper, chopped

2 garlic cloves, minced

2 teaspoons cumin

1 (15-ounce / 425-g) can black beans, drained and rinsed

1 cup cooked brown rice

8 small corn tortillas

Toppings:

1 to 2 slices avocado (optional)

1 to 2 slices tomato (optional)

¼ cup shredded lettuce (optional)

2 tablespoons chopped fresh cilantro (optional)

1. Preheat the oven to 425ºF (220ºC) and line a baking sheet with foil. Spread the sweet potato evenly over the baking sheet, spray with nonstick cooking spray, and roast for 15 to 20 minutes, or until tender.

2. Meanwhile, in a large skillet over medium heat, add the olive oil, onion, bell pepper, and minced garlic. Sauté for 5 to 10 minutes, stirring frequently. Add the cumin and stir well.

3. Add the beans and cooked rice, and sauté for another 5 minutes over medium heat.

4. Add the roasted sweet potato to the rice mixture and stir well, mashing some of the larger pieces of sweet potato if desired.

5. Add the filling to the tortillas along with your desired toppings, and serve immediately.

Per Serving

calories: 301 | fat: 6g | protein: 11g

carbs: 55g | sugars: 1g | fiber: 9g

sodium: 157mg | cholesterol: 0mg

Asparagus and Mushroom Crustless Quiche

1 tablespoon olive oil

1 large yellow or white onion, sliced into half-moons

½ teaspoon freshly ground black pepper

2 cups chopped mushrooms

2 cups chopped asparagus

4 large eggs

4 large egg whites

1 cup nonfat or low-fat milk

½ cup shredded low-fat cheese

1. Preheat the oven to 350ºF (180ºC).

2. Heat the olive oil in a cast iron or ovenproof skillet over medium heat. Add the onion slices and sprinkle with the black pepper. Cook the onions until they are golden brown and starting to caramelize, about 10 minutes.

3. Remove the skillet from the heat and spread the onions evenly across the bottom. Spread the mushrooms and asparagus evenly over the onions.

4. In a medium bowl, add the eggs, egg whites, milk, cheese, and black pepper. Stir with a fork, beating just enough to break up the yolks and white. Pour the custard over the vegetables and onions.

5. Transfer the skillet to the oven, and bake for 45 minutes to 1 hour, until fully cooked and lightly browned across the top. Let the quiche cool for 20 minutes, and then slice into four wedges.

Per Serving

calories: 213 | fat: 11g | protein: 19g

carbs: 12g | sugars: 4g | fiber: 3g

sodium: 256mg | cholesterol: 195mg

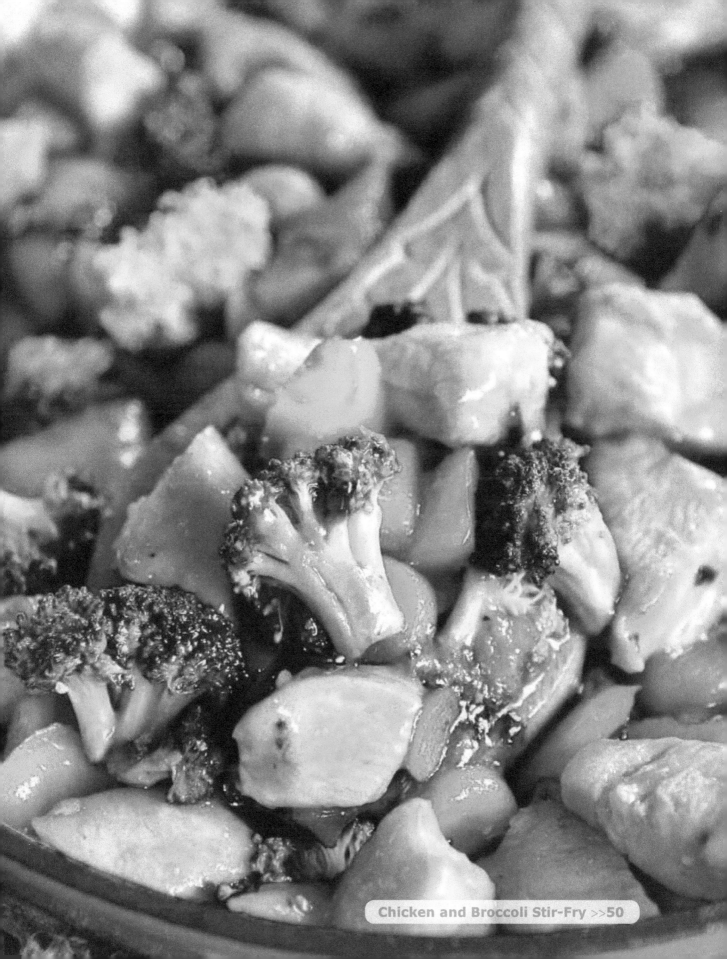

Chicken and Broccoli Stir-Fry >>50

5 POULTRY AND FISH

69 Chicken and Broccoli Stir-Fry

70 Grilled Chicken, Avocado, and Apple Salad

71 Turkey Cutlets with Herbs

72 Balsamic-Roasted Chicken Breasts

73 Chicken Legs with Rice and Peas

74 Spaghetti and Chicken Meatballs

75 Coconut Chicken Curry

76 Mexican-Style Turkey Stuffed Peppers

77 Shrimp Noodle Bowls with Ginger Broth

78 Salmon and Asparagus in Foil

79 Spinach and Feta Salmon Burgers

80 Halibut with Greens and Ginger

81 Baked Flounder Packets with Summer Squash

82 Almond-Crusted Tuna Cakes

83 Pecan-Crusted Catfish

Chicken and Broccoli Stir-Fry

Prep Time: 10 minutes

Cook Time: 15 minutes

Serving: 4

---

2 tablespoons olive oil, divided

2 boneless, skinless chicken breasts, cubed

2 garlic cloves, minced

3 small carrots, thinly sliced

15 ounces (425 g) frozen chopped broccoli florets, thawed

8 ounces (227 g) sliced water chestnuts, drained and thoroughly rinsed

3 tablespoons balsamic vinegar, divided

2 teaspoons ground ginger

1. Heat ½ tablespoon of olive oil in a wok or large sauté pan over medium heat. Add the cubed chicken and cook until lightly browned and cooked through, about 5 to 7 minutes. Transfer chicken to a bowl, cover, and set aside.

2. Add 1½ tablespoons of olive oil to the pan, along with the garlic and carrots. Cook until the carrots begin to soften, about 3 to 4 minutes. Add the thawed broccoli florets and water chestnuts along with 1 tablespoon of balsamic vinegar and cook for 3 to 4 minutes.

3. Add the remaining balsamic vinegar and ground ginger. Add the cooked chicken back in and stir until well combined.

4. Serve over brown rice, if desired.

Per Serving

calories: 189 | fat: 9g | protein: 14g

carbs: 12g | sugars: 3g | fiber: 3g

sodium: 68mg | cholesterol: 33mg

Grilled Chicken, Avocado, and Apple Salad

Prep Time: 15 minutes

Cook Time: 8 minutes

Serving: 4

Cooking spray

2 tablespoons olive oil

3 tablespoons balsamic vinegar

4 (4-ounce / 113-g) skinless, boneless chicken-breast halves

8 cups mixed salad greens

1 cup diced peeled apple

¾ cup avocado, peeled and pitted

Optional: 2 tablespoons freshly squeezed lime juice

1. Prepare a grill for high heat. Apply cooking spray to the grill rack. If you don't have a grill, you can broil the chicken in an oven-safe skillet under the broiler element for 5 to 6 minutes.

2. Combine olive oil, balsamic vinegar, and lime juice (if using) in a small bowl. Place chicken on a large plate. Spoon 2 tablespoons of oil mixture over the chicken, reserving the rest for the salad dressing. Turn chicken to coat, and let stand for 5 minutes.

3. Place chicken on grill rack. Cook for 4 minutes on each side or until an instant-read thermometer registers 165ºF (74ºC). Remove to a plate and cut crosswise into strips.

4. Arrange greens, apple, and avocado on 4 serving plates. Arrange chicken over greens. Drizzle reserved dressing over salads.

Per Serving

calories: 288 | fat: 16g | protein: 27g

carbs: 8g | sugars: 4g | fiber: 5g

sodium: 81mg | cholesterol: 65mg

Turkey Cutlets with Herbs

Prep Time: 5 minutes

Cook Time: 8 minutes

Serving: 4

---

2 tablespoons olive oil

2 lemons, sliced

1 package (approximately 1 pound / 454 g) turkey-breast cutlets (without antibiotics)

½ teaspoon garlic powder

Freshly ground black pepper, to taste

4 cups baby spinach

½ cup water

2 teaspoons dried thyme

1. In a large skillet over medium-high heat, heat the oil.

2. Add about 6 lemon slices to the skillet.

3. Sprinkle the turkey-breast cutlets with garlic powder and black pepper. Place the turkey cutlets into the skillet and cook for about 3 minutes on each side until the turkey is no longer pink, and is slightly browned at the edges. Remove them from the heat and add them to 4 plates.

4. Add the spinach to the pan along with ½ cup of water and steam, stirring frequently for about 2 minutes. Remove the greens and lemons with tongs or a slotted spoon and divide between plates.

5. Serve topped with dried thyme.

Per Serving

calories: 204 | fat: 8g | protein: 30g

carbs: 8g | sugars: 1g | fiber: 4g

sodium: 92mg | cholesterol: 70mg

Balsamic-Roasted Chicken Breasts

Prep Time: 30 minutes

Cook Time: 40 minutes

Serving: 5

¼ cup balsamic vinegar

1 tablespoon olive oil

2 teaspoons dried oregano

2 garlic cloves, minced

⅛ teaspoon salt

½ teaspoon freshly ground black pepper

2 (4-ounce / 113-g) boneless, skinless, chicken-breast halves

Cooking spray

1. In a small bowl, add the vinegar, olive oil, oregano, garlic, salt, and pepper. Mix to combine.

2. Put the chicken in a resealable plastic bag. Pour the vinegar mixture in the bag with the chicken, seal the bag, and coat the chicken to marinate. Refrigerate for 30 minutes.

3. Preheat the oven to 400ºF (205ºC). Spray a small baking dish with cooking spray.

4. Put the chicken in prepared baking dish and pour the marinade over the chicken. Cover and bake for 35 to 40 minutes, or until an instant-read thermometer registers 165ºF (74ºC).

5. Let sit for 5 minutes, then serve with your favorite vegetables.

Per Serving

calories: 226 | fat: 11g | protein: 25g

carbs: 6g | sugars: 0g | fiber: 1g

sodium: 129mg | cholesterol: 65mg

Chicken Legs with Rice and Peas

Prep Time: 5 minutes

Cook Time: 45 minutes

**Serving: 4

4 chicken drumsticks

3 tablespoons olive oil

4 garlic cloves, chopped

1 tablespoon paprika

1 teaspoon dried oregano

1 cup instant brown rice

2¾ cup frozen peas

1. Preheat the oven to 425ºF (220ºC).

2. Place the drumsticks in a 9-by-13-inch baking dish.

3. In a small skillet, heat the olive oil over medium heat. Add the garlic, paprika, and oregano. Cook for 1 minute, and remove from the heat.

4. Pour the mixture over the drumsticks and turn to coat evenly. Bake for about 45 minutes, or until an instant-read thermometer reads 180ºF (82ºC).

5. While the chicken bakes, cook the rice according to the package directions. When the rice has 7 minutes of cook time remaining, stir in the peas and re-cover.

6. Divide the rice among four plates and top each with a drumstick, skin removed.

Per Serving

calories: 345 | fat: 15g | protein: 18g

carbs: 40g | sugars: 2g | fiber: 4g

sodium: 96mg | cholesterol: 48mg

Spaghetti and Chicken Meatballs

2 pounds (907 g) ground chicken

2 large eggs

½ cup panko bread crumbs

1 tablespoon freshly grated Parmesan cheese

1 tablespoon Dijon mustard

½ tablespoon Italian seasoning

½ teaspoon kosher or sea salt

½ teaspoon ground black pepper

⅛ teaspoon crushed red pepper flakes

12 ounces (340 g) whole-grain spaghetti

1 (24-ounce / 680-g) jar lower-sodium marinara sauce

1. Preheat the oven to 375ºF (190ºC). Fit a baking sheet with a wire rack and coat with cooking spray.

2. In a mixing bowl, mix the ground chicken, eggs, bread crumbs, Parmesan cheese, Dijon mustard, Italian seasoning, salt, black pepper, and red pepper flakes until thoroughly combined. Form into 2-inch balls and line up on the wire rack. Bake for 18 to 22 minutes, until the internal temperature reaches 165ºF (74ºC).

3. While the meatballs cook, bring a large pot of water to a boil. Cook the spaghetti according to the package directions.

4. Bring the marinara sauce to a simmer in a pot or a saucepan, stirring frequently. Serve the meatballs over the spaghetti and spoon the marinara sauce on top.

Per Serving

calories: 426 | fat: 15g | protein: 29g

carbs: 40g | sugars: 5g | fiber: 5g

sodium: 394mg | cholesterol: 148mg

Coconut Chicken Curry

Prep Time: 10 minutes

Cook Time: 45 minutes

Serving: 4

---

1 cup brown jasmine rice

2 cups water

2 teaspoons olive oil

2 garlic cloves, minced

2 tablespoons minced fresh ginger

1 tablespoon curry powder

1 medium apple, peel on, cored and diced

1 tablespoon honey

½ cup low-fat/light coconut milk

¾ cup low-sodium chicken broth

1 pound (454 g) boneless, skinless chicken breast, cut into bite-size cubes

¼ cup chopped unsalted cashews

2 tablespoons golden raisins

4 tablespoons chopped fresh cilantro leaves

1. In a medium saucepan with a tight-fitting lid, combine the rice and water, and bring to a boil. Stir once, cover, and reduce heat to low. Simmer for 30 to 35 minutes. Do not lift the lid or stir.

2. Meanwhile, heat the olive oil in a large skillet over medium heat. Add the garlic and sauté for 1 minute. Add the ginger and curry powder and mix well, cooking for 1 minute.

3. Add the apple, honey, coconut milk, and broth, reduce the heat to medium, and cook for about 3 minutes.

4. Add the chicken to the pan, stir all the ingredients, and cover the pan. Simmer over medium-low heat until the chicken is cooked through and an instant-read thermometer registers 165ºF (74ºC), about 30 minutes.

5. Add the cashews and raisins and stir in the cilantro.

6. Fluff the rice with a fork. Serve the chicken over the rice.

Per Serving

calories: 439 | fat: 12g | protein: 31g

carbs: 51g | sugars: 11g | fiber: 4g

sodium: 69mg | cholesterol: 65mg

Mexican-Style Turkey Stuffed Peppers

Prep Time: 15 minutes

Cook Time: 1 hour 10 minutes

Serving: 6

6 red bell peppers, tops cut off

½ cup water

1 tablespoon canola oil

½ yellow onion, peeled and diced

1½ pounds (680 g) ground turkey

4 garlic cloves, peeled and minced

2 tablespoons store-bought low-sodium taco seasoning

2 tablespoons no-salt-added tomato paste

½ teaspoon kosher or sea salt

1 (15-ounce / 425-g) can fire-roasted petite diced tomatoes, drained

1 (15-ounce / 425-g) can black beans, drained and rinsed

1 (4-ounce / 113-g) can diced green chiles

½ cup fresh cilantro leaves, chopped

1 cup shredded Monterey Jack cheese

1. Preheat the oven to 375ºF (190ºC). Coat a baking dish with cooking spray. Place the peppers in the baking dish, pour ½ cup of water into the bottom of the dish, and cover with aluminum foil. Bake for 15 minutes and remove from the oven.

2. Heat the canola oil in a skillet over medium heat. Add the onion and ground turkey. Sauté for 7 to 10 minutes, until the turkey is browned. Stir in the garlic, taco seasoning, tomato paste, and salt. Add the diced tomatoes, black beans, and green chiles and bring to a simmer. Remove from the heat and stir in the cilantro. Taste and adjust the seasoning, if necessary.

3. Place the bell peppers in the baking dish. Fill each with the turkey black bean mixture. Bake uncovered for 35 to 40 minutes, until the peppers are tender. Top with the Monterey Jack cheese and bake for an additional 5 to 10 minutes, until the cheese is bubbly.

4. For leftovers, place in microwaveable airtight containers and reheat in the microwave on high for 2 to 3 minutes, until heated through.

Per Serving

calories: 374 | fat: 15g | protein: 30g

carbs: 27g | sugars: 4g | fiber: 7g

sodium: 528mg | cholesterol: 95mg

Shrimp Noodle Bowls with Ginger Broth

Prep Time: 15 minutes

Cook Time: 35 minutes

Serving: 6

Broth:

1 pound (454 g) shrimp, deveined and divided

2 cups unsalted fish stock

2-inch piece ginger, peeled and sliced

2 teaspoons chili garlic sauce

½ teaspoon kosher or sea salt

½ teaspoon ground black pepper

Noodle Bowls:

8 ounces (227 g) brown rice noodles

1 tablespoon canola oil

½ yellow onion, peeled and thinly sliced

1 red bell pepper, seeded and thinly sliced

1 cup sugar snap peas, thinly sliced

4 garlic cloves, peeled and minced

¼ teaspoon kosher or sea salt

½ cup fresh cilantro leaves (optional)

Make the Broth

1. Peel the shrimp and place the shells in a large pot. Set the peeled shrimp aside. Add the fish stock, ginger, chili garlic sauce, salt, and black pepper to the pot and bring to a simmer for 15 minutes.

Make the Noodle Bowls

2. While the broth is simmering, bring a large pot of water to a boil. Cook the noodles according to the package directions.

3. In that same pot, heat the canola oil to medium. Add the yellow onion, red bell pepper, and snap peas and sauté for 4 to 5 minutes, until the vegetables are slightly soft. Add the shrimp and cook for 2 to 3 minutes, then stir in the garlic and salt.

4. Divide the noodles and shrimp mixture into 6 bowls and pour the broth into each bowl. Top with the cilantro, if desired.

Per Serving

calories: 272 | fat: 5g | protein: 20g

carbs: 36g | sugars: 3g | fiber: 4g

sodium: 430mg | cholesterol: 115mg

Salmon and Asparagus in Foil

5 minutes

Cook Time: 20 minutes

Serving: 4

4 (5-ounce / 142-g) salmon fillets

1 pound (454 g) fresh asparagus, ends trimmed, divided

2 teaspoons dried dill, divided

Freshly squeezed lemon juice

Freshly ground black pepper, to taste (optional)

Lemon wedges, for serving

1. Preheat the oven to 450ºF (235ºC).

2. Prepare four 12-by-18-inch sheets of aluminum foil. Spray the center of each sheet of foil with nonstick cooking spray.

3. Place one salmon fillet in the center of each sheet, top with a quarter of the asparagus, ½ teaspoon of dill, and a squeeze of lemon juice. Sprinkle with black pepper (if using).

4. Bring up the sides of the foil and fold the top over twice. Seal the ends, leaving room for air to circulate inside the packet. Repeat with the remaining fillets.

5. Place the packets on a baking sheet and bake for 15 to 18 minutes, or until the salmon is opaque.

6. Use caution when opening the packets, as the steam is very hot. Serve with lemon wedges on the side.

Per Serving

calories: 202 | fat: 7g | protein: 31g

carbs: 5g | sugars: 0g | fiber: 3g

sodium: 110mg | cholesterol: 63mg

Spinach and Feta Salmon Burgers

Prep Time: 10 minutes

Cook Time: 20 minutes

Serving: 4

1 pound (454 g) salmon fillets, skin removed

1 cup fresh spinach, chopped

½ cup panko bread crumbs

¼ cup crumbled feta cheese

1 large egg

1 tablespoon Dijon mustard

½ teaspoon dried dill

¼ teaspoon kosher or sea salt

¼ teaspoon ground black pepper

½ cup plain nonfat Greek yogurt

½ English cucumber, sliced

1 beefsteak tomato, sliced

1. Preheat the oven to 400ºF (205ºC). Line a baking sheet with parchment paper.

2. Place the salmon in the bowl of a food processor and pulse until ground. Transfer to a bowl and stir in the spinach, bread crumbs, feta cheese, egg, Dijon mustard, dill, salt, and black pepper until well combined. Use your hands to form 4 burger-size patties. Place them on the parchment paper and bake for 20 minutes, until the internal temperature reaches 145ºF (63ºC).

3. Serve the burgers with dollops of the Greek yogurt and slices of the cucumber and tomato.

4. For leftovers, place the burgers in microwaveable airtight containers for up to 3 to 4 days. Reheat in the microwave on high for 2 to 3 minutes, until heated through. Assemble the burgers before consuming.

Per Serving

calories: 238 | fat: 8g | protein: 30g

carbs: 10g | sugars: 3g | fiber: 1g

sodium: 453mg | cholesterol: 109mg

Halibut with Greens and Ginger

---

4 (4-ounce / 113-g) halibut fillets, rinsed and patted dry

½ teaspoon freshly ground black pepper

3 teaspoons olive oil, divided

4 cups baby spinach

1 tablespoon minced peeled ginger

2 garlic cloves, minced

1 tablespoon balsamic vinegar

1 tablespoon freshly squeezed lime juice

1. Sprinkle the fish with the black pepper. Using your fingertips, gently press in the seasoning so it adheres to the fish.

2. In a large nonstick skillet, heat 2 teaspoons of the olive oil over medium-high heat, swirling to coat the bottom. Cook the fish for 2 minutes, or until browned on the bottom. Turn over, and cook for 2 minutes more, or until the fish flakes easily when tested with a fork. Transfer to a plate and cover to keep warm.

3. In the same skillet, heat the remaining 1 teaspoon of olive oil, swirling the bottom to coat. Add the spinach, ginger, and garlic, and cook, stirring constantly, for 2 minutes, or until the spinach begins to wilt. Remove the skillet from the heat.

4. Add the balsamic vinegar and lime juice to the spinach and stir. Divide the spinach among four plates and top each serving with a halibut fillet. Serve immediately.

Per Serving

calories: 162 | fat: 6g | protein: 24g

carbs: 3g | sugars: 0g | fiber: 1g

sodium: 84mg | cholesterol: 35mg

Baked Flounder Packets with Summer Squash

Prep Time: 5 minutes

Cook Time: 10 minutes

Serving: 4

4 (6-ounce / 170-g) flounder fillets, or other white fish

Freshly ground black pepper, to taste

2 medium zucchini, sliced into thin rounds

2 medium yellow summer squash, sliced into thin rounds

1 medium red onion, sliced

2 tablespoons olive oil

2 tablespoons freshly squeezed lemon juice

1 lemon, thinly sliced

2 teaspoons dried basil

1. Preheat the oven to 450ºF (235ºC). Prepare four 12-by-18-inch sheets of aluminum foil. Spray the center of each sheet of foil with nonstick cooking spray.

2. Season the fish with the black pepper. Place one fish fillet on each piece of foil.

3. Arrange the zucchini, squash, and onion slices around each fillet. Drizzle ½ tablespoon of olive oil and ½ tablespoon of lemon juice onto the vegetables and fish.

4. Arrange a few lemon slices on top of each fillet and top each piece with ½ teaspoon of dried basil.

5. Bring up the sides of the foil and fold the tops over twice. Seal the ends, leaving room for air to circulate inside the packet. Set the packets on a rimmed baking sheet, and bake for 8 minutes. Carefully open one packet to check the fish and test with a fork to see if it flakes easily.

6. Serve immediately, using caution when opening the packets as the steam will be very hot.

Per Serving

calories: 233 | fat: 9g | protein: 32g

carbs: 10g | sugars: 3g | fiber: 4g

sodium: 130mg | cholesterol: 98mg

Almond-Crusted Tuna Cakes

Prep Time: 15 minutes

Cook Time: 15 minutes

Serving: 4

½ cup almonds

9 ounces (255 g) canned albacore tuna

2 large eggs

½ cup panko bread crumbs

¼ cup fresh parsley leaves, chopped

Zest and juice of ½ lemon

1 tablespoon Dijon mustard

1 teaspoon Italian seasoning

¼ teaspoon kosher or sea salt

¼ teaspoon ground black pepper

2 tablespoons olive oil

1. Place almonds in a food processor and pulse until crumbly. Transfer to a shallow dish.

2. Clean the food processor. Put the tuna, eggs, bread crumbs, parsley, lemon zest and juice, Dijon mustard, Italian seasoning, salt, and black pepper in the food processor and pulse until a paste forms, scraping down the sides of the processor bowl as needed. Form the mixture into 4 cakes. Press the patties into the crushed almonds on all sides.

3. Heat the olive oil in a skillet over medium heat. Place the cakes in the hot oil and fry for 3 minutes on each side, until browned and crispy.

4. For leftovers, place in microwaveable airtight containers for 3 to 4 days. Reheat in the microwave on high for 1 to 2 minutes, until heated through.

Per Serving

calories: 293 | fat: 19g | protein: 20g

carbs: 11g | sugars: 1g | fiber: 3g

sodium: 435mg | cholesterol: 124mg

Pecan-Crusted Catfish

Prep Time: 5 minutes

Cook Time: 20 minutes

Serving: 4

4 catfish fillets (approximately 1 pound / 454 g)

½ teaspoon freshly ground black pepper

½ teaspoon garlic powder

2 teaspoons dried rosemary

2 egg whites, beaten

¾ cup pecans, chopped

Lemon wedges for serving

1. Preheat the oven to 400ºF (205ºC).

2. Line a baking sheet with foil and coat the foil with nonstick cooking spray.

3. Sprinkle the catfish fillets with the black pepper, garlic, and rosemary, then dip each fillet into the egg whites to coat.

4. Place the chopped pecans on a plate and press the egg-coated fillets firmly into the pecans, turning to coat both sides. Place the fillets on the baking sheet.

5. Bake for 20 minutes or until the fish flakes easily with a fork.

6. Serve with lemon wedges and enjoy.

Per Serving

calories: 263 | fat: 20g | protein: 18g

carbs: 4g | sugars: 1g | fiber: 3g

sodium: 228mg | cholesterol: 47mg

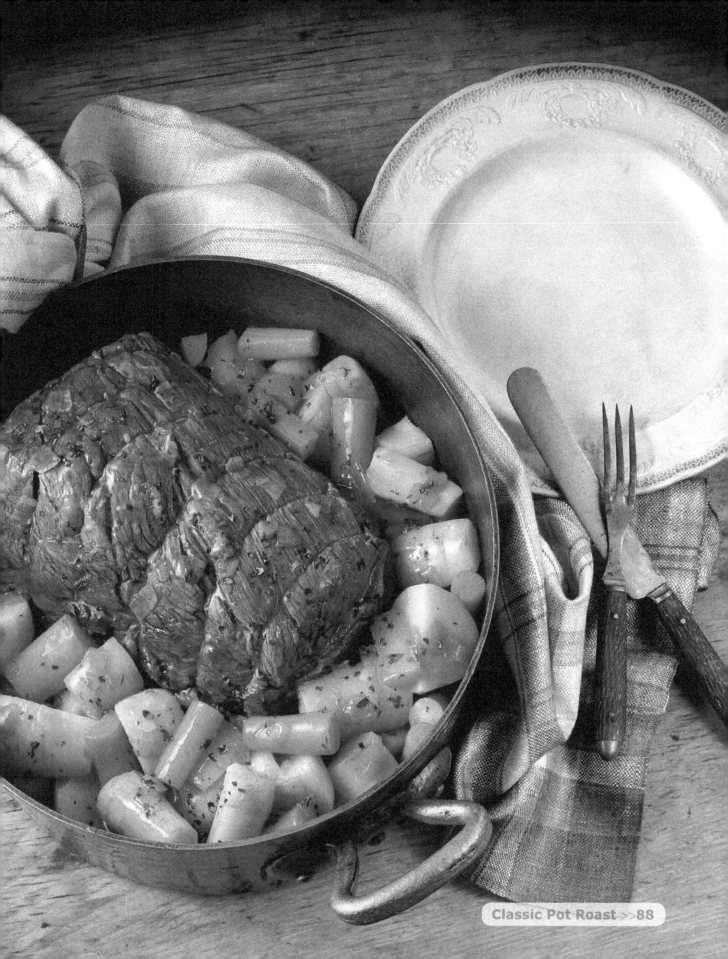

Classic Pot Roast >>88

6 BEEF AND PORK

86 Steak Tacos

87 Grilled Flank Steak with Peach Compote

88 Classic Pot Roast

89 Slow Cooker Beef Ragu with Polenta

90 Beef Tenderloin with Balsamic Tomatoes

91 Herb-Roasted Pork Loin and Potatoes

92 Tuscan Pork Kebabs

93 Pork and Vegetable Stew

94 Mustard-Crusted Pork Tenderloin

95 Apple-Cinnamon Baked Pork Chops

Steak Tacos

Prep Time: 15 minutes

Cook Time: 13 minutes

Serving: 4

1 pound (454 g) beef flank (or round) steak

1 teaspoon chili powder

1 teaspoon olive oil

1 green bell pepper, cored and coarsely chopped

1 red onion, coarsely chopped

8 (6-inch) corn tortillas, warm

2 tablespoons freshly squeezed lime juice

Optional for serving:
1 avocado, sliced, and coarsely chopped cilantro

1. Rub the steak with chili powder (and salt and pepper, if desired).

2. Heat olive oil in a large skillet over medium-high heat.

3. Add steak and cook for 6 to 8 minutes on each side or until it reaches your desired degree of doneness. Remove from heat.

4. Place steak on a plate and cover with aluminum foil. Let rest for 5 minutes.

5. Add the bell pepper and onion to skillet. Cook on medium heat, stirring frequently, for 3 to 5 minutes or until onion is translucent. Remove from heat.

6. Cut steak against the grain into thin slices.

7. Top tortillas evenly with beef, onion mixture, and lime juice. Garnish with avocado and cilantro, if using.

8. Serve immediately.

Per Serving

calories: 358 | fat: 12g | protein: 28g

carbs: 34g | sugars: 0g | fiber: 2g

sodium: 139mg | cholesterol: 40mg

Grilled Flank Steak with Peach Compote

Prep Time: 15 minutes

Cook Time: 25 minutes

Serving: 6

Peach Compote:

2 peaches, cored and diced

1 tablespoon honey

½ tablespoon apple cider vinegar

¼ teaspoon ground cinnamon

¼ teaspoon ground ginger

¼ teaspoon ground nutmeg

¼ teaspoon kosher or sea salt

Grilled Flank Steak:

1½ pounds (680 g) flank steak

2 tablespoons canola oil

½ teaspoon kosher or sea salt

¼ teaspoon ground black pepper

Make the Peach Compote

1. Place the peaches, honey, apple cider vinegar, cinnamon, ginger, nutmeg, and salt in a saucepan and bring to a simmer. Stirring frequently, cook for 7 to 10 minutes, until the peaches are tender and the mixture has thickened. Remove from the heat and reserve.

Make the Grilled Flank Steak

2. Heat a grill or grill pan over medium-high heat. Coat the steak with the canola oil, salt, and black pepper. Grill for 4 to 6 minutes per side, until the internal temperature reaches 155ºF (68ºC). Let rest for 5 to 10 minutes on a cutting board, then thinly slice across the grain. Divide the steak and serve with the peach compote.

Per Serving

calories: 236 | fat: 12g | protein: 24g

carbs: 7g | sugars: 5g | fiber: 1g

sodium: 356mg | cholesterol: 45mg

Classic Pot Roast

Prep Time: 20 minutes

Cook Time: 3½ to 4 hours

Serving: 8

2 tablespoons canola oil

2 pounds (907 g) beef chuck roast

1 teaspoon kosher or sea salt

½ teaspoon ground black pepper

1 large yellow onion, peeled and sliced

4 cloves garlic, peeled

2 cups unsalted beef stock

½ cup dry red wine (optional)

2 bay leaves

5 fresh thyme sprigs

4 Yukon Gold or red potatoes, cubed

2 carrots, peeled and sliced

1. Heat the canola oil in a Dutch oven or stockpot over medium heat. Season the roast with the salt and black pepper. Sear it in the oil for 3 to 4 minutes on all sides, until it has a brown crust.

2. Add the onion and garlic to the pot, then the beef stock and red wine (if using). Bring to a simmer. Add the bay leaves and thyme sprigs. Place the lid on the pot and cook for 3 to 4 hours, until the meat is tender. During the last 30 minutes of the cooking process, add the potatoes and carrots to the pot. Taste and adjust the seasoning, if necessary. Remove the bay leaves and thyme sprigs before serving.

Per Serving

calories: 320 | fat: 12g | protein: 33g

carbs: 17g | sugars: 2g | fiber: 2g

sodium: 430mg | cholesterol: 82mg

Slow Cooker Beef Ragu with Polenta

Prep Time: 20 minutes

Cook Time: 4 to 8 hours

Serving: 8

Slow Cooker Beef Ragu:

2 tablespoons canola oil

2 pounds (907 g) beef chuck roast, fat trimmed

½ teaspoon kosher or sea salt

½ teaspoon ground black pepper

1 yellow onion, peeled and sliced

4 garlic cloves, peeled and minced

1 (32-ounce / 907-g) can no-salt-added crushed tomatoes

1 tablespoon dried oregano leaves

2 bay leaves

Creamy Polenta:

4 cups water or unsalted vegetable or chicken stock

1 cup coarse-ground yellow cornmeal

½ teaspoon kosher or sea salt

1 tablespoon olive oil or unsalted butter

¼ cup freshly grated Parmesan cheese

Make the Slow Cooker Beef Ragu

1. Heat the canola oil in a large skillet over medium-high heat. Season the chuck roast with the salt and black pepper. Sear the chuck roast in the hot oil for 2 to 3 minutes per side, until a brown crust forms. Transfer the chuck roast to the bowl of a slow cooker. Add the onion, garlic, tomatoes, dried oregano, and bay leaves to the slow cooker. Cook on low for 6 to 8 hours or high for 3 to 4 hours, until the beef shreds easily with a fork. Turn off the slow cooker, discard the bay leaves, and shred all of the beef. Reserve with the lid on until ready to use.

Make the Creamy Polenta

2. When the beef ragu has about 30 minutes left to cook, start making the polenta. Place the water or stock in a large saucepan and bring to a boil. Slowly whisk in the cornmeal and reduce the heat to a slow simmer. Cook the polenta for 30 minutes, whisking occasionally, until the liquid has been absorbed and the polenta is creamy.

3. Remove from the heat and whisk in the salt, olive oil or butter, and Parmesan cheese.

4. To serve, add a spoonful of the polenta to a large bowl and top with a hearty scoop of the beef ragu.

5. For leftovers, store in microwaveable airtight containers up to 5 days. Reheat in the microwave on high for 2 to 3 minutes, until heated through.

Per Serving

calories: 343 | fat: 15g | protein: 34g

carbs: 19g | sugars: 4g | fiber: 3g

sodium: 434mg | cholesterol: 85mg

Beef Tenderloin with Balsamic Tomatoes

Prep Time: 5 minutes

Cook Time: 20 minutes

Serving: 2

½ cup balsamic vinegar

¾ cup coarsely chopped, seeded tomato

2 teaspoons olive oil

2 (3- to 4-ounce / 85- to 113-g, ¾-inch-thick) beef tenderloin steaks, trimmed of visible fat

1 teaspoon fresh thyme (or ½ teaspoon dried)

1. In a small saucepan, bring the balsamic vinegar to a boil. Reduce the heat and simmer, uncovered, for 5 minutes, or until the liquid is reduced to ¼ cup. Stir in the tomatoes and cook for 1 to 2 minutes more. Remove the saucepan from the heat.

2. In a large skillet, heat the olive oil over medium-high heat. Add the steaks, and reduce the heat to medium. Cook the steaks to desired doneness, turning once. Allow 7 to 9 minutes per side for medium (160ºF / 71ºC).

3. Spoon the balsamic tomatoes over the steaks, and sprinkle with the thyme. Serve immediately.

Per Serving

calories: 298 | fat: 20g | protein: 17g

carbs: 11g | sugars: 0g | fiber: 1g

sodium: 69mg | cholesterol: 58mg

Herb-Roasted Pork Loin and Potatoes

Prep Time: 5 minutes

Cook Time: 1 hour

Serving: 4

1 (1-pound / 454-g) pork loin, trimmed

8 garlic cloves

¼ cup olive oil, divided

Freshly ground black pepper, to taste

1 cup cubed raw sweet potato

1 cup small gold potatoes, quartered

8 fresh thyme sprigs, chopped

1. Preheat the oven to 350ºF (180ºC). Rub the pork with the garlic and 2 tablespoons of the olive oil. Season with the black pepper. Coat a 9-by-13-inch baking dish with nonstick cooking spray.

2. Place the pork in the prepared baking dish. Bake for approximately 60 minutes, or until an instant-read thermometer inserted in the center registers 145ºF (63ºC).

3. Twenty minutes into the cooking time, place the cubed and sliced sweet potatoes and gold potatoes on a rimmed baking dish, drizzle with the remaining olive oil, sprinkle with the thyme, and place in the oven. The potatoes should be finished roasting about the same time as the pork and should be tender and slightly browned.

4. Once the pork is finished cooking, remove from the oven and let the meat stand for 15 minutes before carving. Cut into eight slices. Serve with the roasted potatoes and a green salad.

Per Serving

calories: 426 | fat: 22g | protein: 27g

carbs: 21g | sugars: 3g | fiber: 4g

sodium: 56mg | cholesterol: 45mg

Tuscan Pork Kebabs

Prep Time: 15 minutes

Cook Time: 10 minutes

Serving: 4

4 teaspoons olive oil, plus 1 tablespoon

1 tablespoon lemon zest

½ teaspoon freshly ground black pepper

2 garlic cloves, crushed

1 pound (454 g) pork tenderloin, trimmed and cut into 1-inch pieces

16 (1-inch) pieces red bell pepper

16 button mushrooms

8 cups chopped, stemmed spinach

Per Serving

calories: 251 | fat: 14g | protein: 24g

carbs: 11g | sugars: 4g | fiber: 3g

sodium: 88mg | cholesterol: 45mg

1. Prepare the grill to medium-high heat, or preheat the broiler to high, for at least 5 minutes.

2. Combine 4 teaspoons of the olive oil, lemon zest, black pepper, and garlic in a large bowl, stirring well. Add the pork, and marinate at room temperature for 15 minutes, tossing occasionally.

3. Thread the pork, bell peppers, and mushrooms alternately onto each of the eight 8-inch skewers. Place the skewers on a grill rack coated with cooking spray, and grill, turning occasionally, for 10 minutes, or until the pork is no longer pink and is completely cooked. If using the broiler, place the skewers under the broiler and cook for 5 minutes, or until the edges begin to brown, then rotate and cook for an additional 5 minutes.

4. While the pork cooks, heat a large skillet over medium-high heat. Add 1 tablespoon of the olive oil to the pan, and swirl to coat. Add the spinach and sauté for 5 minutes until the spinach wilts.

5. Serve the spinach alongside the kebabs.

Pork and Vegetable Stew

Prep Time: 10 minutes

Cook Time: 35 minutes

Serving: 4

2 tablespoons olive oil

1 medium onion, chopped

1 pound (454 g) pork tenderloin, cut into thin strips

4 carrots, thinly sliced

2 teaspoons dried thyme

4 garlic cloves, minced

2 red potatoes, cubed

½ cup low-sodium chicken stock

1. Heat the olive oil in a large nonstick skillet over medium heat. Add the onion and cook for 5 to 7 minutes, or until the onions are translucent.

2. Add the pork and continue cooking for 10 minutes. Add the carrots, thyme, and garlic, and cook for another 5 minutes.

3. Add the potatoes and chicken stock and cover with a lid. Bring to a boil and simmer for 10 to 15 minutes, stirring occasionally until the potatoes are cooked through, the flavors have blended, and the pork is cooked through and no longer pink. Pork tenderloin should be cooked to an internal temperature of 145°F (63°C) to 160°F (71°C).

4. Serve immediately.

Per Serving

calories: 289 | fat: 12g | protein: 22g

carbs: 24g | sugars: 3g | fiber: 4g

sodium: 89mg | cholesterol: 45mg

Mustard-Crusted Pork Tenderloin

15 minutes

15 minutes

3 tablespoons Dijon mustard

3 tablespoons honey

1 teaspoon dried rosemary

1 tablespoon olive oil

1 pound (454 g) pork tenderloin

Salt and freshly ground black pepper, to taste

1. Preheat the oven to 425ºF (220ºC) with the rack set in the middle. In a small bowl, combine the Dijon mustard, honey, and rosemary. Stir to combine, set aside.

2. Preheat an oven-safe skillet over high heat and add the olive oil. While it is heating up, pat pork loin dry with a paper towel and season lightly with salt and pepper on all sides. When the skillet is hot, sear the pork loin on all sides until golden brown, about 3 minutes per side. Remove from the heat and spread honey-mustard mixture evenly to coat the pork loin.

3. Place the skillet in the oven and cook the pork loin for 15 minutes, or until an instant-read thermometer registers 145ºF (63ºC).

4. Remove from the oven and allow to rest for 3 minutes. Slice the pork into ½-inch slices and serve.

Per Serving

calories: 220 | fat: 9g | protein: 19g

carbs: 14g | sugars: 13g | fiber: 0g

sodium: 307mg | cholesterol: 45mg

Apple-Cinnamon Baked Pork Chops

Prep Time: 10 minutes

Cook Time: 40 minutes

Serving: 4

2 apples, peeled, cored, and sliced

1 teaspoon ground cinnamon, divided

4 boneless pork chops (½-inch thick)

Salt and freshly ground black pepper, to taste

¾ cup water

2 tablespoons pure maple syrup

1 tablespoon olive oil

1. Preheat the oven to 375ºF (190ºC). Layer apples in bottom of casserole dish. Sprinkle with ½ teaspoon of cinnamon.

2. Trim fat from the pork chops. Lay chops on top of the apple slices. Sprinkle with a dash of salt and pepper.

3. In a small bowl, combine ¾ cup of water, maple syrup, and remaining cinnamon. Pour the mixture over the chops. Drizzle the chops with 1 tablespoon of olive oil.

4. Bake uncovered in preheated oven for 30 to 45 minutes or until an instant-read thermometer registers between 145ºF (63ºC) and 160ºF (71ºC). Allow to rest for 3 minutes before serving.

Per Serving

calories: 244 | fat: 10g | protein: 21g

carbs: 22g | sugars: 19g | fiber: 4g

sodium: 254mg | cholesterol: 45mg

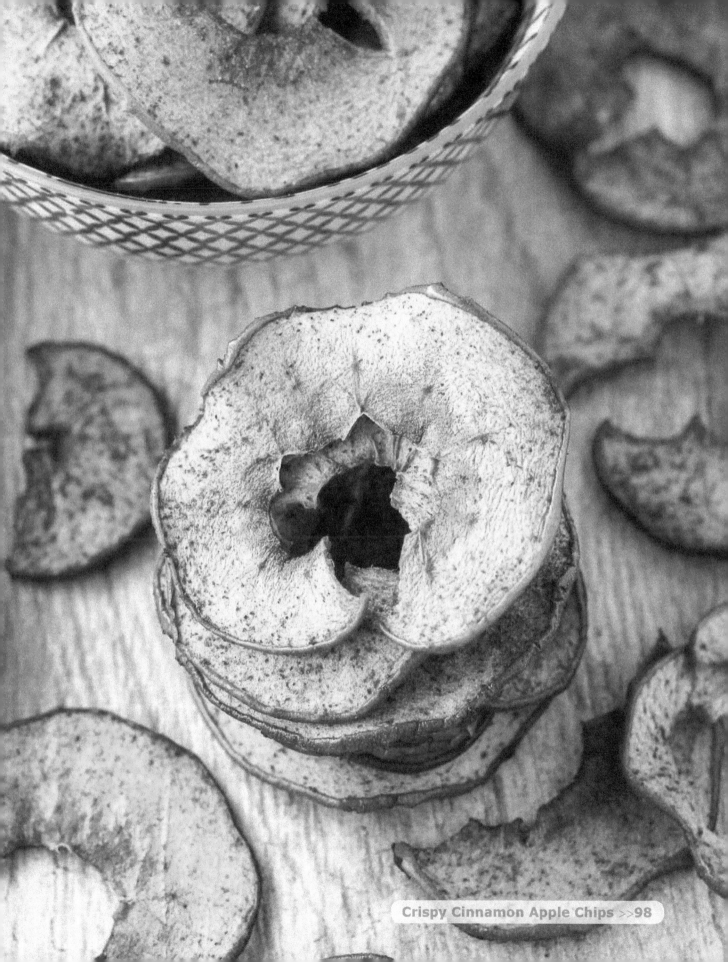

Crispy Cinnamon Apple Chips >>98

7 SNACKS, SIDES, AND DESSERTS

98 Crispy Cinnamon Apple Chips

99 Root Vegetable Chips with Yogurt Dip

100 Peanut Butter Blondies

101 Pumpkin Pie Snack Bars

102 Cauliflower Mashed "Potatoes"

103 Roasted Brussels Sprouts

104 Broccoli with Garlic and Lemon

105 Brown-Rice Pilaf

106 Grilled Corn and Edamame Succotash

107 Rosemary Roasted Beets and Carrots

108 Peanut Butter Rice Pudding

109 Single-Serve Cherry-Vanilla Cupcake

110 Chocolate Mint "Ice Cream"

110 Classic Hummus

111 Chunky Black-Bean Dip

111 Stovetop Cheese Popcorn

Crispy Cinnamon Apple Chips

Prep Time: 15 minutes

Cook Time: 1¼ to 1½ hours

Serving: 4

3 apples, thinly sliced crosswise, seeded

1 tablespoon ground cinnamon

1 teaspoon granulated sugar

¼ teaspoon kosher salt

1. Preheat the oven to 275ºF (135ºC). Coat a baking sheet with cooking spray.

2. In a large bowl, whisk together the cinnamon, sugar, and salt. Add the apple slices and toss to evenly coat. Line up the apple slices on the baking sheet and roast for 45 minutes, then flip each chip and roast for another 45 minutes, until dried and crispy.

3. Once cooled, store in an airtight container or plastic bag for up to 7 days.

Per Serving

calories: 80 | fat: 0g | protein: 0g

carbs: 21g | sugars: 15g | fiber: 4g

sodium: 147mg | cholesterol: 0mg

Root Vegetable Chips with Yogurt Dip

Cook Time: 20 minutes

Serving: 6

Roasted Root Vegetable Chips:

1 sweet potato

1 Yukon Gold potato

1 beet

3 tablespoons canola oil

¼ teaspoon kosher salt

French Onion Yogurt Dip:

1 tablespoon canola oil

1 yellow onion, peeled and thinly sliced

3 cloves garlic, peeled and minced

1 cup nonfat plain Greek yogurt

1 tablespoon mayonnaise

1 teaspoon Worcestershire sauce

½ teaspoon ground black pepper

½ teaspoon onion powder

¼ teaspoon kosher or sea salt

¼ teaspoon dried mustard powder

⅛ teaspoon ground cayenne pepper

Make the Roasted Root Vegetable Chips

1. Preheat the oven to 425ºF (220ºC). Coat a large baking sheet with cooking spray.

2. Thinly slice the sweet potato, Yukon Gold potato, and beet with a mandoline. Be careful! Coat them in the canola oil and sprinkle with the salt. Roast for about 16 minutes, flipping after 8 minutes, until crispy and lightly browned.

Make the French Onion Yogurt Dip

3. Heat the canola oil in a skillet over medium-low heat. Add the onion and sauté for 8 to 10 minutes, until caramelized and brown. Stir in the garlic and cook until fragrant, about 1 minute. Transfer the mixture to a bowl and add the Greek yogurt, mayonnaise, Worcestershire sauce, black pepper, onion powder, salt, dried mustard powder, and cayenne pepper. Mix until combined.

4. The chips are best when served immediately. The sauce will keep in the refrigerator for 5 days.

Per Serving

calories: 168 | fat: 11g | protein: 5g

carbs: 13g | sugars: 5g | fiber: 1g

sodium: 266mg | cholesterol: 2mg

Peanut Butter Blondies

Prep Time: 10 minutes

Cook Time: 30 minutes

Makes 9 blondies

1 (15-ounce / 425-g) can chickpeas, rinsed and drained

½ cup powdered peanut butter

¼ cup rolled oats

¼ cup unsweetened vanilla cashew milk

¼ cup canned unsweetened pumpkin purée

¼ cup granulated no-calorie sweetener

2 tablespoons no-sugar-added creamy peanut butter

2 teaspoons vanilla extract

¾ teaspoon baking powder

⅛ teaspoon baking soda

¼ teaspoon salt

2 tablespoons mini chocolate chips (optional)

1. Preheat the oven to 350ºF (180ºC). Lightly coat an 8 × 8-inch baking pan with cooking spray.

2. In a food processor, combine the chickpeas, powdered peanut butter, oats, cashew milk, pumpkin, sweetener, creamy peanut butter, vanilla, baking powder, baking soda, and salt. Pulse a few times to break up the beans, then process until you get a smooth paste, 1 to 2 minutes.

3. Scrape the batter into the pan and smooth out the top with a spatula. If you are using the optional chips, place them on top.

4. Transfer to the oven and bake until a toothpick inserted into the center comes out clean and the top is lightly browned, about 25 minutes.

5. Remove the blondies from the oven and allow to cool in the pan, then cut into 9 squares. Enjoy immediately or store in an airtight container in the refrigerator for up to 1 week.

Per Serving

calories: 104 | fat: 3g | protein: 6g

carbs: 13g | sugars: 2g | fiber: 4g

sodium: 120mg | cholesterol: 0mg

Pumpkin Pie Snack Bars

Prep Time: 5 minutes

Cook Time: 35 minutes

Makes 8 squares

2 scoops vanilla pea protein powder

½ cup coconut flour

½ cup granulated no-calorie sweetener

¹/₃ cup oat flour

1 tablespoon flaxseed meal

2 teaspoons pumpkin pie spice

½ teaspoon ground mace

¾ teaspoon baking soda

¼ teaspoon salt

¾ cup fat-free milk

1 (15-ounce / 425-g) can unsweetened pumpkin purée

1. Preheat the oven to 325ºF (163ºC). Line a 9 × 9-inch baking pan with parchment paper.

2. In a large bowl, whisk together the pea protein, coconut flour, sweetener, oat flour, flaxseed meal, pumpkin pie spice, mace, baking soda, and salt. Add the milk and pumpkin purée and mix until completely blended (it will be like a moist dough).

3. Spread into the prepared pan, smoothing the top. Transfer to the oven and bake until the edges begin to brown and the top appears dry, 30 to 35 minutes.

4. Remove from the oven and cool completely in the pan on a wire rack, then refrigerate until cold. Remove from the refrigerator and lift the parchment to remove from the pan. Cut into 16 squares.

Per Serving

calories: 104 | fat: 2g | protein: 8g

carbs: 14g | sugars: 3g | fiber: 5g

sodium: 203mg | cholesterol: 1mg

Cauliflower Mashed "Potatoes"

Prep Time: 10 minutes

Cook Time: 10 minutes

Serving: 4

16 cups water (enough to cover cauliflower)

1 head cauliflower (about 3 pounds / 1.4 kg), trimmed and cut into florets

4 garlic cloves

1 tablespoon olive oil

¼ teaspoon salt

⅛ teaspoon freshly ground black pepper

2 teaspoons dried parsley

1. Bring a large pot of water to a boil. Add the cauliflower and garlic. Cook for about 10 minutes or until the cauliflower is fork tender. Drain, return it back to the hot pan, and let it stand for 2 to 3 minutes with the lid on.

2. Transfer the cauliflower and garlic to a food processor or blender. Add the olive oil, salt, and pepper, and purée until smooth.

3. Taste and adjust the salt and pepper. Remove to a serving bowl and add the parsley and mix until combined.

4. Garnish with additional olive oil, if desired. Serve immediately.

Per Serving

calories: 87 | fat: 4g | protein: 4g

carbs: 12g | sugars: 0g | fiber: 5g

sodium: 210mg | cholesterol: 0mg

Roasted Brussels Sprouts

Prep Time: 5 minutes

Cook Time: 20 minutes

Serving: 4

1½ pounds (680 g) Brussels sprouts, trimmed and halved

2 tablespoons olive oil

¼ teaspoon salt

½ teaspoon freshly ground black pepper

1. Preheat the oven to 400ºF (205ºC).

2. Combine the Brussels sprouts and olive oil in a large mixing bowl and toss until they are evenly coated.

3. Turn the Brussels sprouts out onto a large baking sheet and flip them over so they are cut-side down with the flat part touching the baking sheet. Sprinkle with salt and pepper.

4. Bake for 20 to 30 minutes or until the Brussels sprouts are lightly charred and crisp on the outside and toasted on the bottom. The outer leaves will be extra dark, too.

5. Serve immediately.

Per Serving

calories: 134 | fat: 8g | protein: 6g

carbs: 15g | sugars: 4g | fiber: 7g

sodium: 189mg | cholesterol: 0mg

Broccoli with Garlic and Lemon

Prep Time: 2 minutes

Cook Time: 4 minutes

Serving: 4

---

1 cup water

4 cups broccoli florets

1 teaspoon olive oil

1 tablespoon minced garlic

1 teaspoon lemon zest

Salt and freshly ground
black pepper, to taste

1. In a small saucepan, bring 1 cup of water to a boil. Add the broccoli to the boiling water and cook for 2 to 3 minutes or until tender, being careful not to overcook. The broccoli should retain its bright-green color. Drain the water from the broccoli.

2. In a small sauté pan over medium-high heat, add the olive oil. Add the garlic and sauté for 30 seconds. Add the broccoli, lemon zest, salt, and pepper. Combine well and serve.

Per Serving

calories: 38 | fat: 1g | protein: 3g

carbs: 5g | sugars: 0g | fiber: 3g

sodium: 24mg | cholesterol: 0mg

Brown-Rice Pilaf

Prep Time: 5 minutes

Cook Time: 10 minutes

Serving: 4

1 cup low-sodium vegetable broth

½ tablespoon olive oil

1 clove garlic, minced

1 scallion, thinly sliced

1 tablespoon minced onion flakes

1 cup instant brown rice

⅛ teaspoon freshly ground black pepper

1. Mix the vegetable broth, olive oil, garlic, scallion, and minced onion flakes in a saucepan and bring to a boil.

2. Add rice, return mixture to boil, then reduce heat and simmer for 10 minutes.

3. Remove from heat and let stand for 5 minutes.

4. Fluff with a fork and season with black pepper.

Per Serving

calories: 100 | fat: 2g | protein: 2g

carbs: 19g | sugars: 1g | fiber: 2g

sodium: 35mg | cholesterol: 0mg

Grilled Corn and Edamame Succotash

Prep Time: 10 minutes

Cook Time: 10 minutes

Serving: 4

---

4 ears sweet corn, husked

3 tablespoons olive oil, divided

2 cups shelled edamame

1 pint cherry tomatoes, halved

Zest and juice of 1 lime

¼ cup chopped fresh cilantro

2 tablespoons chopped fresh basil

¼ teaspoon kosher or sea salt

¼ teaspoon ground black pepper

1. Preheat the grill over medium heat. Coat the corn in a teaspoon of the olive oil and grill for about 10 minutes, turning every couple of minutes. Let cool and cut the kernels from the cob.

2. Place the corn kernels, edamame, and cherry tomatoes in a large bowl. Next, add the remaining olive oil, lime zest and juice, cilantro, basil, salt, and black pepper. Stir to combine, and serve with your favorite summer-inspired entrée.

Per Serving

calories: 163 | fat: 17g | protein: 17g

carbs: 32g | sugars: 6g | fiber: 10g

sodium: 163mg | cholesterol: 0mg

Rosemary Roasted Beets and Carrots

Prep Time: 5 minutes

Cook Time: 35 minutes

Serving: 4

1½ pounds (680 g) beets, peeled and cut into ½-inch wedges

1 pound (454 g) carrots, scrubbed and cut into 2-inch pieces

1/3 cup red wine vinegar

2 tablespoons olive oil

2 fresh rosemary sprigs

¼ teaspoon freshly ground black pepper

1. Preheat the oven to 450ºF (235ºC).

2. In a large bowl, combine all of the ingredients, and toss to evenly coat the vegetables.

3. Spread the vegetables on a rimmed baking sheet and roast, tossing once, for 30 to 35 minutes, or until the vegetables are tender.

4. Serve immediately.

Per Serving

calories: 180 | fat: 8g | protein: 4g

carbs: 27g | sugars: 17g | fiber: 8g

sodium: 211mg | cholesterol: 0mg

Peanut Butter Rice Pudding

1 cup uncooked brown rice

2½ cups nonfat milk

¼ cup unsalted natural peanut butter

²/₃ cup water

2 teaspoons pure vanilla extract

1 tablespoon honey (more or less to taste)

1. In a medium saucepan, combine the rice and milk, and bring to a boil.

2. Lower to a simmer and cover. Simmer, covered, for 20 to 40 minutes, or until rice is thick and fluffy. (Length of time depends on the variety of brown rice used.)

3. Stir in the peanut butter and water and return to a boil. Remove from the heat. Allow to sit, covered, for 15 to 20 minutes, or until the water is absorbed.

4. Stir in the vanilla and honey.

5. Enjoy warm or cold.

Per Serving

calories: 262 | fat: 9g | protein: 9g

carbs: 35g | sugars: 10g | fiber: 3g

sodium: 92mg | cholesterol: 2mg

Single-Serve Cherry-Vanilla Cupcake

Prep Time: 3 minutes

Cook Time: 3½ to 4 minutes

Serving: 1

¼ cup oat flour or whole-wheat pastry flour

3 packets (1½ teaspoons) stevia

¼ teaspoon baking powder

Pinch of salt

¼ teaspoon coconut oil

2 tablespoons nonfat (0%) plain Greek yogurt

2 tablespoons fat-free milk

1 large egg white or 2 tablespoons liquid egg whites

½ teaspoon vanilla extract

4 cherries, diced

1. Lightly coat a 10-ounce (283-g) or larger mug or ramekin with cooking spray.

2. In a small bowl, whisk together the flour, stevia, baking powder, and salt. In a separate bowl, whisk together the coconut oil, yogurt, milk, egg white(s), and vanilla. Fold in the cherries. Gradually mix in the dry ingredients until just incorporated.

3. Pour the batter into the prepared mug or ramekin and microwave for 3½ minutes, then check to see if it's set. If needed, add an additional 30 seconds. (Note that because microwaves vary in their power level, always start with the minimum time, then check and continue cooking if necessary.)

4. Immediately run a knife around the edges to help separate the cake from the mug. Firmly place a plate over the mug, flip the mug over, and gently shake the mug to release the cake onto the plate.

5. Let cool for 5 minutes.

Per Serving

calories: 180 | fat: 2g | protein: 11g

carbs: 30g | sugars: 6g | fiber: 5g

sodium: 237mg | cholesterol: 2mg

Chocolate Mint "Ice Cream"

3 bananas, sliced and frozen

4 tablespoons unsweetened cocoa powder

½ teaspoon peppermint extract

2 to 3 tablespoons nonfat or low-fat milk (optional)

Prep Time: 10 minutes

Cook Time: 0 minutes

Serving: 4

1. Remove the frozen bananas from the freezer and let stand for about 5 minutes.

2. Add the banana, cocoa, and peppermint extract to a food processor and pulse until the banana slices are finely chopped. Then purée until the mixture resembles soft-serve ice cream, adding the milk (if using).

Per Serving

calories: 92 | fat: 1g | protein: 2g

carbs: 23g | sugars: 11g | fiber: 4g

sodium: 2mg | cholesterol: 0mg

Classic Hummus

1 (15-ounce / 425-g) can chickpeas, drained and rinsed

3 tablespoons sesame tahini

2 tablespoons olive oil

3 garlic cloves, chopped

Juice of 1 lemon

Salt and freshly ground black pepper, to taste

Prep Time: 5 minutes

Cook Time: 0 minutes

Serving: 6 to 8

1. In a food processor or blender, combine all the ingredients until smooth but thick. Add water if necessary to produce a smoother hummus.

2. Store covered for up to 5 days.

Per Serving

calories: 147 | fat: 10g | protein: 6g

carbs: 11g | sugars: 0g | fiber: 4g

sodium: 64mg | cholesterol: 0mg

Chunky Black-Bean Dip

1 (15-ounce / 425-g) can black beans, drained, with liquid reserved

½ (7-ounce / 198-g) can chipotle peppers in adobo sauce

¼ cup plain Greek yogurt

Freshly ground black pepper, to taste

Prep Time: 5 minutes

Cook Time: 0 minutes

Serving: 6 to 8

1. Combine beans, peppers, and yogurt in a food processor or blender and process until smooth. Add some of the bean liquid, 1 tablespoon at a time, for a thinner consistency.
2. Season to taste with black pepper.
3. Serve.

Per Serving

calories: 70 | fat: 1g | protein: 5g

carbs: 11g | sugars: 0g | fiber: 4g

sodium: 159mg | cholesterol: 0mg

Stovetop Cheese Popcorn

¼ cup canola oil

½ cup white or yellow popcorn kernels

3 tablespoons nutritional yeast

½ teaspoon kosher salt

Prep Time: 10 minutes

Cook Time: 20 minutes

Makes 15 cups

1. Heat the canola oil over medium-high heat in a large stockpot. Add the popcorn kernels and place a lid on the pot. Let cook, shaking the pot periodically, until the popping stops. Remove from the heat, transfer to a large bowl, and top with the nutritional yeast and salt, shaking the bowl to coat the hot popcorn.

Per Serving

calories: 54 | fat: 4g | protein: 1g

carbs: 5g | sugars: 0g | fiber: 1g

sodium: 77mg | cholesterol: 0mg

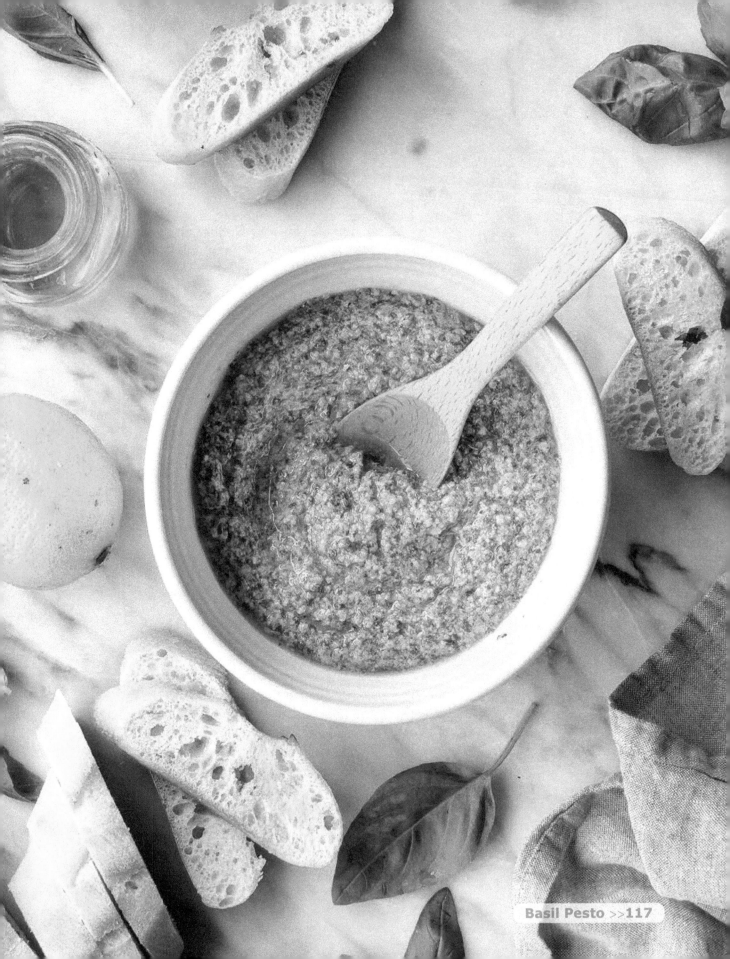

8 BROTHS, CONDIMENTS, AND SAUCES

114 Potato Vegetable Broth

115 Homemade Chicken Broth

116 Red Pepper Pesto

117 Basil Pesto

118 Simple Tomato Sauce

119 Creamy Spinach-Artichoke Sauce

120 Greek Yogurt Mayonnaise

120 Chili Lime Marinade

121 Fresh Vegetable Salsa

121 Honey Chipotle Sauce

122 Tzatziki Sauce

122 Creamy Avocado "Alfredo" Sauce

Potato Vegetable Broth

Prep Time: 15 minutes

Cook Time: 30 minutes

Makes 10 cups

---

2 pounds (907 g) potatoes, scrubbed, peeled, and cut into 1-inch pieces

4 large leeks, white parts only, split, well-rinsed, and sliced

2 medium carrots, scrubbed and cut into 1-inch pieces

½ teaspoon freshly ground black pepper

1 bay leaf

1 teaspoon dried thyme

1. In a heavy-bottomed stockpot, combine all of the ingredients. Add about 8 cups of water or more as needed to completely cover the vegetables.

2. Bring to a boil, reduce heat, cover, and simmer for 30 minutes.

3. Pass the broth through a large sieve or colander, pressing on the vegetables to extract as much juice as possible. Discard the vegetable pulp.

4. Store in the refrigerator in an airtight container for four to five days. Use it generously as needed in your favorite recipes.

Per Serving

calories: 10 | fat: 0g | protein: 1g

carbs: 2g | sugars: 0g | fiber: 0g

sodium: 29mg | cholesterol: 0mg

Homemade Chicken Broth

Prep Time: 15 minutes

Cook Time: 2 hours

Makes 8 cups

---

4 quarts cold water

1 (3-pound / 1.4-kg) whole chicken (or chicken parts, such as wings and breasts)

4 celery stalks with leaves, trimmed and cut into 2-inch pieces

4 medium carrots, peeled and cut into 2-inch pieces

1 medium onion, peeled and quartered

1 medium potato, peeled and quartered

6 garlic cloves

1 small bunch parsley

1 teaspoon dried thyme

2 bay leaves

1. In a large stockpot, combine all of the ingredients, and bring to a boil over medium-high heat. Reduce the heat to medium-low and simmer, partially covered, until the chicken is falling apart, about 2 hours.

2. Strain the broth through a large sieve or colander into a large bowl. Use a wooden spoon to press on the solids to extract as much of the broth as possible. Save the chicken meat if desired or discard along with the vegetable pulp and bones.

3. Allow the broth to cool in the bowl or divide the broth among several shallow containers to cool it quickly.

4. Cover loosely and refrigerate overnight. Use a spoon to remove the fat that congeals on the surface before using.

Per Serving

calories: 86 | fat: 3g | protein: 6g

carbs: 9g | sugars: 1g | fiber: 0g

sodium: 50mg | cholesterol: 7mg

Red Pepper Pesto

Prep Time: 20 minutes

Cook Time: 10 minutes

Makes 3 cups

4 red bell peppers, tops sliced off and deseeded

3 cups fresh basil leaves

3 tablespoons cashews

3 tablespoons grated Parmesan cheese

1 tablespoon olive oil

3 garlic cloves

¼ teaspoon salt

1. Place peppers in the oven on a sheet pan and turn broiler to high. Broil until peppers have blackened on all sides, turning a few times, for about 10 minutes total.

2. Remove peppers from heat and place in a bowl. Cover with plastic wrap and set aside to cool.

3. Peel the cooled peppers. In a food processor, combine peeled peppers with the remaining ingredients. Process until mixture is smooth and resembles a pesto.

Per Serving (¼ cup)

calories: 50 | fat: 3g | protein: 2g

carbs: 5g | sugars: 0g | fiber: 1g

sodium: 74mg | cholesterol: 0mg

Basil Pesto

Prep Time: 15 minutes

Cook Time: 5 minutes

Makes 3½ cups

1 cup fresh basil leaves

1 cup fresh baby spinach leaves

½ cup freshly grated Parmesan cheese

½ cup olive oil

¼ cup pine nuts

4 garlic cloves, peeled

¼ teaspoon kosher or sea salt

¼ teaspoon ground black pepper

1. Place all the ingredients in the bowl of a food processor and process until a paste forms, scraping down the sides of the bowl with a spatula as needed. Taste and adjust the seasoning, if necessary.

2. Place leftovers in airtight containers and refrigerate for up to 5 days, or freeze pesto in an airtight container for up to 2 months and thaw as needed. Or divide pesto into cube trays, seal in a plastic bag, and freeze for up to 2 months. Pop pesto cubes out of the ice cube tray as needed.

Per Serving (½ cup)

calories: 209 | fat: 20g | protein: 4g

carbs: 2g | sugars: 0g | fiber: 1g

sodium: 231mg | cholesterol: 0mg

Simple Tomato Sauce

Prep Time: 5 minutes

Cook Time: 1 hour

Makes 4 cups

1 tablespoon olive oil

1 cup minced yellow onion

4 garlic cloves, minced

1 (28-ounce / 794-g) can no-salt crushed tomatoes

¼ cup water

2 tablespoons no-salt added tomato paste

2 tablespoons honey

2 tablespoons oregano

1 tablespoon basil

½ teaspoon crushed red pepper flakes

1. In a large pot over medium heat, heat the olive oil. Add the onion and garlic and cook for 3 to 5 minutes, or until tender. Reduce the heat to low.

2. Add the remaining ingredients, and cover. Cook over low heat for 50 to 60 minutes.

3. Taste to adjust seasonings.

4. Serve hot as you would store-bought tomato sauce. Store any leftovers in an airtight container in the refrigerator for up to one week.

Per Serving (½ cup)

calories: 71 | fat: 2g | protein: 2g

carbs: 13g | sugars: 5g | fiber: 2g

sodium: 16mg | cholesterol: 0mg

Creamy Spinach-Artichoke Sauce

Prep Time: 5 minutes

Cook Time: 15 minutes

Makes 3 cups

---

2 teaspoons extra-virgin olive oil

4 cloves garlic, minced

½ cup diced onion

1 tablespoon whole-wheat flour

1 cup fat-free milk

½ cup shredded part-skim Mozzarella cheese (2 ounces / 57 g)

½ cup nonfat (0%) plain Greek yogurt

2 ounces (57 g) ⅓-less-fat cream cheese

10 ounces (283 g) frozen chopped spinach, thawed and squeezed of excess water

1 (14-ounce / 397-g) can water-packed artichoke hearts, rinsed, drained, and chopped

¼ cup grated Parmesan cheese

¼ teaspoon salt

½ teaspoon freshly ground black pepper

½ teaspoon red pepper flakes

¼ teaspoon grated lemon zest

1. In a large skillet, heat the olive oil over medium heat. Add the garlic and onion and cook until softened, 3 to 4 minutes. Add the flour and stir until the flour begins to brown. Stir in the milk and bring to a boil, then immediately reduce the heat to low and simmer for 3 to 4 minutes, until it starts to thicken.

2. Add the Mozzarella, Greek yogurt, and cream cheese and stir until melted, 2 to 3 minutes. Add the spinach and artichoke hearts and cook stirring constantly for 3 to 4 minutes to warm through.

3. Add the Parmesan, salt, black pepper, pepper flakes, and lemon zest and cook until the cheese has melted and the ingredients are thoroughly combined, an additional 2 to 3 minutes.

4. Serve immediately or refrigerate in a covered container for 3 to 4 days.

Per Serving (⅓ cup)

calories: 104 | fat: 4g | protein: 8g

carbs: 11g | sugars: 3g | fiber: 5g

sodium: 244mg | cholesterol: 9mg

Greek Yogurt Mayonnaise

6 ounces (170 g) nonfat or low-fat plain Greek yogurt

1 teaspoon apple cider vinegar

¼ teaspoon yellow mustard

¼ teaspoon hot sauce

¼ teaspoon freshly ground black pepper

¼ teaspoon paprika

¼ teaspoon salt

Prep Time: 2 minutes

Cook Time: 0 minutes

Serving: 2

1. Mix all the ingredients together and blend well. Adjust seasonings to suit taste.

Per Serving

calories: 8 | fat: 0g | protein: 1g

carbs: 1g | sugars: 1g | fiber: 0g

sodium: 65mg | cholesterol: 0mg

Chili Lime Marinade

¼ cup canola oil

Zest and juice of 1 lime

2 tablespoons apple cider vinegar

1 tablespoon chili powder

1 teaspoon garlic powder

1 teaspoon onion powder

¼ teaspoon kosher or sea salt

¼ teaspoon ground black pepper

Prep Time: 10 minutes

Cook Time: 0 minutes

Serving: 2

1. Whisk all the ingredients together, and store in an airtight container in the refrigerator for up to 5 days or freeze it for up to 2 months.

Per Serving

calories: 300 | fat: 16g | protein: 8g

carbs: 37g | sugars: 17g | fiber: 10g

sodium: 125mg | cholesterol: 0mg

Fresh Vegetable Salsa

2 cups cored and diced bell peppers

2 cups diced tomatoes

1 cup diced zucchini

½ cup chopped red onion

¼ cup freshly squeezed lime juice

2 garlic cloves, minced

1 teaspoon freshly ground black pepper

¼ teaspoon salt

Prep Time: 10 minutes

Cook Time: 0 minutes

Serving: 2

1. Wash the vegetables and prepare as directed.

2. In a large bowl, combine all the ingredients. Toss gently to mix.

3. Cover and refrigerate for at least 30 minutes to allow the flavors to blend.

Per Serving (¼ cup)

calories: 10 | fat: 0g | protein: 0g

carbs: 2g | sugars: 1g | fiber: 1g

sodium: 26mg | cholesterol: 0mg

Honey Chipotle Sauce

1 tablespoon chopped chipotle chiles in adobo sauce

3 tablespoons honey

3 tablespoons no-salt-added tomato paste

3 tablespoons unsalted vegetable or chicken stock

2½ tablespoons white wine vinegar

Prep Time: 10 minutes

Cook Time: 15 minutes

Serving: 2

1. Pour all the ingredients into a small saucepan and bring to a simmer for about 15 minutes, until slightly thickened.

2. Store in an airtight container in the refrigerator for up to 7 days.

Per Serving (¼ cup)

calories: 136 | fat: 0g | protein: 1g

carbs: 32g | sugars: 30g | fiber: 2g

sodium: 124mg | cholesterol: 0mg

Tzatziki Sauce

1 medium English cucumber, seeded

1½ cups plain low-fat Greek yogurt

2 small garlic cloves, minced

1 teaspoon freshly squeezed lemon juice

Dash freshly ground black pepper

2 tablespoons finely chopped fresh mint or dill

Prep Time: 5 minutes

Cook Time: 0 minutes

Makes 2 cups

1. Coarsely grate the cucumber into a medium bowl, and drain off the excess liquid.
2. Add the yogurt, garlic, lemon juice, black pepper, and mint or dill. Mix well.
3. Refrigerate to chill for about an hour before serving.

Per Serving (1 tablespoon)

calories: 10 | fat: 0g | protein: 1g

carbs: 1g | sugars: 1g | fiber: 0g

sodium: 4mg | cholesterol: 1mg

Creamy Avocado "Alfredo" Sauce

1 ripe avocado, peeled and pitted

1 tablespoon dried basil

1 clove garlic

1 tablespoon lemon juice

1 tablespoon olive oil

⅛ teaspoon salt

Prep Time: 10 minutes

Cook Time: 0 minutes

Serving: 4

1. Add the avocado, basil, garlic clove, lemon juice, olive oil, and salt to a food processor. Blend until a smooth, creamy sauce forms.
2. Pour the sauce over hot pasta or vegetable noodles.

Per Serving

calories: 104 | fat: 10g | protein: 1g

carbs: 4g | sugars: 0g | fiber: 3g

sodium: 43mg | cholesterol: 0mg

Appendix 1 Measurement Conversion Chart

DAYS	BREAKFAST	LUNCH	DINNER	SNACK/DESSERT
1	Apricot-Banana Breakfast Barley [14]	Curried Roasted Cauliflower and Lentil Salad [30]	Pasta Primavera [63]	Crispy Cinnamon Apple Chips [98]
2	Strawberry Orange Beet Smoothie [24]	Loaded Baked Sweet Potatoes [51]	Turkey Cutlets with Herbs [71]	Stovetop Cheese Popcorn [111]
3	Blueberry-Oatmeal Muffin in a Mug [15]	Cauliflower "Fried Rice" and Mixed Vegetables [58]	Black Bean and Beet Burger [46]	Single-Serve Cherry-Vanilla Cupcake [109]
4	Creamy Peach Quinoa [16]	Shrimp Noodle Bowls with Ginger Broth [77]	Asparagus and Mushroom Crustless Quiche [66]	Chunky Black-Bean Dip [111]
5	Green Apple Pie Protein Smoothie [25]	Coconut Rice and White Beans [53]	Halibut with Greens and Ginger [80]	Peanut Butter Rice Pudding [108]
6	Banana-Almond Pancakes for One [17]	Southwestern Chicken Salad [31]	Herbed Mushroom Rice [62]	Root Vegetable Chips with Yogurt Dip [99]
7	Peach Avocado Smoothie [26]	Pork and Vegetable Stew [93]	Penne with White Beans and Tomatoes [64]	Classic Hummus [110]
8	High-Protein Apple Carrot Hemp Muffins [18]	Cauliflower Butternut Squash Mac and Cheese [54]	Grilled Flank Steak with Peach Compote [87]	Chocolate Mint "Ice Cream" [110]
9	Morning Glory Smoothie [27]	Rustic Tomato Panzanella Salad [32]	Mustard-Crusted Pork Tenderloin [94]	Crispy Cinnamon Apple Chips [98]
10	Egg and Vegetable Breakfast Mug [19]	Steak Tacos [86]	Sweet Potato and Black Bean Wraps [65]	Peanut Butter Blondies [100]

11	Sweet Potato and Black Bean Hash [21]	Bean Pasta with Arugula Avocado Walnut Pesto [55]	Salmon and Asparagus in Foil [78]	Stovetop Cheese Popcorn [111]
12	Almond Butter Banana Chocolate Smoothie [26]	Creamy Butternut Squash Soup [38]	Balsamic-Roasted Chicken Breasts [72]	Single-Serve Cherry-Vanilla Cupcake [109]
13	Egg in a "Pepper Hole" with Avocado [22]	French Lentil Salad with Parsley [36]	Hearty Lentil Soup [50]	Chunky Black-Bean Dip [111]
14	Strawberry Orange Beet Smoothie [24]	Chicken and Broccoli Stir-Fry [69]	Roasted Beet, Avocado, and Watercress Salad [35]	Pumpkin Pie Snack Bars [101]
15	Apricot-Banana Breakfast Barley [14]	Lentil-Walnut Mushroom Tacos [57]	Spinach and Feta Salmon Burgers [79]	Root Vegetable Chips with Yogurt Dip [99]
16	Greek Breakfast Scramble [23]	Cauliflower "Fried Rice" and Mixed Vegetables [58]	White Beans with Spinach and Tomatoes [52]	Classic Hummus [110]
17	Morning Glory Smoothie [27]	Quinoa and Spinach Power Salad [37]	Coconut Chicken Curry [75]	Peanut Butter Blondies [100]
18	Creamy Peach Quinoa [16]	Mushroom and Sweet Potato Mini Quiches [59]	Herb-Roasted Pork Loin and Potatoes [91]	Chocolate Mint "Ice Cream" [110]
19	High-Protein Apple Carrot Hemp Muffins [18]	Pecan-Crusted Catfish [83]	Spinach and Artichoke Grilled Cheese [45]	Pumpkin Pie Snack Bars [101]
20	Peach Avocado Smoothie [26]	Creamy Tomato and Greens Soup [40]	Baked Flounder Packets with Summer Squash [81]	Root Vegetable Chips with Yogurt Dip [99]
21	Banana-Almond Pancakes for One [17]	Chipotle Chicken and Caramelized Onion Panini [44]	Pasta Primavera [63]	Peanut Butter Rice Pudding [108]

Appendix 2 Measurement Conversion Chart

VOLUME EQUIVALENTS(DRY)

US STANDARD	METRIC (APPROXIMATE)
1/8 teaspoon	0.5 mL
1/4 teaspoon	1 mL
1/2 teaspoon	2 mL
3/4 teaspoon	4 mL
1 teaspoon	5 mL
1 tablespoon	15 mL
1/4 cup	59 mL
1/2 cup	118 mL
3/4 cup	177 mL
1 cup	235 mL
2 cups	475 mL
3 cups	700 mL
4 cups	1 L

VOLUME EQUIVALENTS(LIQUID)

US STANDARD	US STANDARD (OUNCES)	METRIC (APPROXIMATE)
2 tablespoons	1 fl.oz.	30 mL
1/4 cup	2 fl.oz.	60 mL
1/2 cup	4 fl.oz.	120 mL
1 cup	8 fl.oz.	240 mL
1 1/2 cup	12 fl.oz.	355 mL
2 cups or 1 pint	16 fl.oz.	475 mL
4 cups or 1 quart	32 fl.oz.	1 L
1 gallon	128 fl.oz.	4 L

TEMPERATURES EQUIVALENTS

FAHRENHEIT(F)	CELSIUS(C) (APPROXIMATE)
225 °F	107 °C
250 °F	120 °C
275 °F	135 °C
300 °F	150 °C
325 °F	160 °C
350 °F	180 °C
375 °F	190 °C
400 °F	205 °C
425 °F	220 °C
450 °F	235 °C
475 °F	245 °C
500 °F	260 °C

WEIGHT EQUIVALENTS

US STANDARD	METRIC (APPROXIMATE)
1 ounce	28 g
2 ounces	57 g
5 ounces	142 g
10 ounces	284 g
15 ounces	425 g
16 ounces (1 pound)	455 g
1.5 pounds	680 g
2 pounds	907 g

Appendix 3 The Dirty Dozen and Clean Fifteen

The Environmental Working Group (EWG) is a nonprofit, nonpartisan organization dedicated to protecting human health and the environment Its mission is to empower people to live healthier lives in a healthier environment. This organization publishes an annual list of the twelve kinds of produce, in sequence, that have the highest amount of pesticide residue-the Dirty Dozen-as well as a list of the fifteen kinds ofproduce that have the least amount of pesticide residue-the Clean Fifteen.

THE DIRTY DOZEN

- **The 2016 Dirty Dozen includes the following produce. These are considered among the year's most important produce to buy organic:**

Strawberries	Spinach
Apples	Tomatoes
Nectarines	Bell peppers
Peaches	Cherry tomatoes
Celery	Cucumbers
Grapes	Kale/collard greens
Cherries	Hot peppers

- *The Dirty Dozen list contains two additional itemskale/collard greens and hot peppers-because they tend to contain trace levels of highly hazardous pesticides.*

THE CLEAN FIFTEEN

- **The least critical to buy organically are the Clean Fifteen list. The following are on the 2016 list:**

Avocados	Papayas
Corn	Kiw
Pineapples	Eggplant
Cabbage	Honeydew
Sweet peas	Grapefruit
Onions	Cantaloupe
Asparagus	Cauliflower
Mangos	

- *Some of the sweet corn sold in the United States are made from genetically engineered (GE) seedstock. Buy organic varieties of these crops to avoid GE produce.*

Appendix 4 Recipe Index

A

Almond Butter Banana Chocolate Smoothie 26
Almond Butter Tofu and Roasted Asparagus 60
Almond-Crusted Tuna Cakes 82
Apple-Cinnamon Baked Pork Chops 95
Apricot-Banana Breakfast Barley 14
Asparagus and Mushroom Crustless Quiche 66
Avocado Egg Salad 34

B

Baked Flounder Packets with Summer Squash 81
Balsamic-Roasted Chicken Breasts 72
Banana-Almond Pancakes for One 17
Barley Soup with Asparagus and Mushrooms 42
Basil Pesto 117
Bean Pasta with Arugula Avocado Walnut Pesto 55
Beef Tenderloin with Balsamic Tomatoes 90
Black Bean and Beet Burger 46
Blueberry-Oatmeal Muffin in a Mug 15
Broccoli with Garlic and Lemon 104
Brown-Rice Pilaf 105
Cauliflower "Fried Rice" and Mixed Vegetables 58

C-D

Cauliflower Butternut Squash Mac and Cheese 54
Cauliflower Mashed "Potatoes" 102
Chicken and Broccoli Stir-Fry 69
Chicken Legs with Rice and Peas 73
Chili Lime Marinade 120
Chipotle Chicken and Caramelized Onion Panini 44
Chocolate Mint "Ice Cream" 110
Chunky Black-Bean Dip 111
Classic Hummus 110
Classic Pot Roast 88
Coconut Chicken Curry 75
Coconut Rice and White Beans 53
Creamy Avocado "Alfredo" Sauce 122
Creamy Butternut Squash Soup 38
Creamy Peach Quinoa 16
Creamy Spinach-Artichoke Sauce 119

Creamy Tomato and Greens Soup 40
Crispy Cinnamon Apple Chips 98
Curried Roasted Cauliflower and Lentil Salad 30

E-F

Egg and Vegetable Breakfast Mug 19
Egg in a "Pepper Hole" with Avocado 22
French Lentil Salad with Parsley 36
Fresh Vegetable Salsa 121

G

Greek Breakfast Scramble 23
Greek Yogurt Mayonnaise 120
Greek Yogurt Oat Pancakes 20
Green Apple Pie Protein Smoothie 25
Grilled Chicken, Avocado, and Apple Salad 70
Grilled Corn and Edamame Succotash 106
Grilled Flank Steak with Peach Compote 87

H

Halibut with Greens and Ginger 80
Hearty Lentil Soup 50
Herb-Roasted Pork Loin and Potatoes 91
Herbed Mushroom Rice 62
High-Protein Apple Carrot Hemp Muffins 18
Homemade Chicken Broth 115
Honey Chipotle Sauce 121

L

Lentil Sloppy Joes 56
Lentil-Walnut Mushroom Tacos 57
Loaded Baked Sweet Potatoes 51

M

Mediterranean Chickpea Tuna Salad 33
Mexican-Style Turkey Stuffed Peppers 76
Morning Glory Smoothie 27
Mushroom and Sweet Potato Mini Quiches 59
Mustard-Crusted Pork Tenderloin 94

P

Pasta Primavera 63
Peach Avocado Smoothie 26
Peanut Butter Blondies 100
Peanut Butter Rice Pudding 108
Pecan-Crusted Catfish 83
Penne with White Beans and Tomatoes 64
Pork and Vegetable Stew 93

Potato Vegetable Broth 114
Pumpkin Pie Snack Bars 101

Q-R

Quick and Easy Black Bean Soup 39
Quinoa and Spinach Power Salad 37
Red Pepper Pesto 116
Roasted Beet, Avocado, and Watercress Salad 35
Roasted Brussels Sprouts 103
Root Vegetable Chips with Yogurt Dip 99
Rosemary Roasted Beets and Carrots 107
Rustic Tomato Panzanella Salad 32

S

Salmon and Asparagus in Foil 78
Shrimp Noodle Bowls with Ginger Broth 77
Simple Tomato Sauce 118
Single-Serve Cherry-Vanilla Cupcake 109
Slow Cooker Beef Ragu with Polenta 89
Southwest Tofu Scramble 49
Southwestern Chicken Salad 31
Spaghetti and Chicken Meatballs 74
Spicy Bean Chili 61
Spinach and Artichoke Grilled Cheese 45
Spinach and Feta Salmon Burgers 79
Steak Tacos 86
Stovetop Cheese Popcorn 111
Strawberry Orange Beet Smoothie 24
Sweet Potato and Black Bean Hash 21
Sweet Potato and Black Bean Wraps 65

T

Turkey Cutlets with Herbs 71
Tuscan Pork Kebabs 92
Two-Potato Cauliflower Soup 43
Tzatziki Sauce 122

W

White Bean Soup with Roasted Eggplant 41
White Beans with Spinach and Tomatoes 52

References

Mayo Clinic Staff. (2019, May 08). DASH diet: Healthy eating to lower your blood pressure. Mayo Clinic. https://www.mayoclinic.org/healthy-lifestyle/nutrition-and-healthy-eating/in-depth/dash-diet/art-20048456

Shirani, Fatemeh. (2013, March 06). Effects of Dietary Approaches to Stop Hypertension (DASH) diet on some risk for developing type 2 diabetes: a systematic review and meta-analysis on controlled clinical trials. National Library of Medicine. https://pubmed.ncbi.nlm.nih.gov/23473733/

L.j. Appel. (1997, April 17). A clinical trial of the effects of dietary patterns on blood pressure. DASH Collaborative Research Group. National Library of Medicine. https://pubmed.ncbi.nlm.nih.gov/9099655/

F. M. Sacks. (1999, July 22). A dietary approach to prevent hypertension: a review of the Dietary Approaches to Stop Hypertension (DASH) Study. National Library of Medicine. https://pubmed.ncbi.nlm.nih.gov/10410299/

CPSIA information can be obtained
at www.ICGtesting.com
Printed in the USA
BVHW061151290621
610723BV00006B/1744